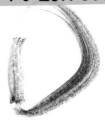

DR. NEAL BARNARD'S
P R O G R A M   F O R
REVERSING
DIABETES

DR. NEAL BARNARD'S
PROGRAM FOR
REVERSING DIABETES

| THE SCIENTIFICALLY
PROVEN SYSTEM FOR
REVERSING DIABETES
WITHOUT DRUGS |

NEAL D. BARNARD, MD
With Menus and Recipes by
Bryanna Clark Grogan

RODALE
wellness

Live happy. Be healthy. Get inspired.

Sign up today to get exclusive access to our authors, exclusive bonuses,
and the most authoritative, useful, and cutting-edge information on health,
wellness, fitness, and living your life to the fullest.

Visit us online at RodaleWellness.com

Join us at RodaleWellness.com/Join

First published in hardcover by Rodale Inc. in December 2006.

First published in paperback by Rodale Inc. in February 2008.

© 2017, 2008, 2006 by Neal D. Barnard, MD

Rodale books may be purchased for business or promotional use or for special sales. For
information, please e-mail: BookMarketing@Rodale.com.

Printed in the United States of America

Rodale Inc. makes every effort to use acid-free ♾, recycled paper ♻.

Book design by Christopher Rhoads

Library of Congress Cataloging-in-Publication Data is on file with the publisher.

ISBN 978–1–63565–127–0

Distributed to the trade by Macmillan

2 4 6 8 10 9 7 5 3 1 paperback

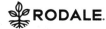

RODALE.

Follow us @RodaleBooks on

We inspire health, healing, happiness, and love in the world.
Starting with you.

This book is dedicated to the memory of my father, Donald M. Barnard, MD, a kind and wise physician, and to the participants in our research studies. I am deeply grateful for your important contribution to this work.

"Dr. Barnard's solid scientific work...represents a major turning point in the treatment and outcome of diabetes. Revolutionary in its implications and spectacular in its clarity, this book—with its simple, safe dietary approach—will bring hope to millions."

—**Hans Diehl, DrHSc, MPH, FACN, chairman of the Lifestyle Medicine Institute in Loma Linda, California, and director of the International Nutrition Research Foundation**

"Dr. Barnard's superb book shows us the numerous advantages of following his nutritional program."

—**William C. Roberts, MD, editor in chief of the *American Journal of Cardiology* and executive director of the Baylor Heart and Vascular Institute in Dallas**

"A promising alternative dietary approach in the treatment of diabetes."

—**William E. Connor, MD, professor of medicine and clinical nutrition at Oregon Health and Science University in Portland**

CONTENTS

ACKNOWLEDGMENTS

I would like to thank the many doctors, nurses, dietitians, and people with diabetes who used the first edition of this book and shared their experiences along the way. They have underscored the power of this approach and the great need for it at a time when the causes of diabetes and the nutritional approach to it remain only dimly understood by a surprisingly large number of caregivers and patients.

The research that culminated in this book was a team effort. I especially want to express my deepest appreciation to the research volunteers who put up with many early mornings, late nights, and needlesticks in performing an important public service. You have taught me a great deal and helped our research immeasurably.

I greatly appreciate the support of the National Institute of Diabetes and Digestive and Kidney Diseases of the National Institutes of Health, particularly Sanford Garfield, PhD, and of the Diabetes Action Education and Research Foundation and its director, Pat DeVoe, RN, BSN, without which our initial research on diabetes would not have been possible. Thank you also to GEICO for allowing us to test this approach in the work setting in cities across the US and to the American Diabetes Association for the opportunity to share our findings along the way.

Joshua Cohen, MD, of the division of endocrinology at George Washington University, was instrumental in planning and guiding our research work. David J. A. Jenkins, MD, PhD, DSc, of the University of Toronto, is an extraordinary mentor whose generosity with his time, knowledge, and ideas is something I hope to pass on to other investigators.

Caroline Trapp, DNP, ANP-BC, CDE, FAANP, has applied this approach in extraordinary ways in her clinical work and in her innovative programs with Native Americans and, along with Meghan Jardine,

MS, MBA, RDN, LD, CDE, has educated and empowered thousands of caregivers.

Susan Levin, MS, RD, Francesca Valente, Rosendo Flores, Jill Eckart, Suruchi Mishra, PhD, Joseph Gonzales, RD, Gabrielle Turner-McGrievy, PhD, RD, and Lisa Gloede, RD, CDE, helped extensively in research planning and in guiding our research participants toward more healthful ways of eating. Brent Jaster, MD; Amber A. Green, RD; Kim Seidl, MS, RD; Trulie Ankerberg-Nobis, RD; Dulcie Ward, RD; Jennifer Reilly, RD; and Mary Ellen Wolfe, RN, CDE, and Robyn Webb shared their expertise and guidance with me and our research participants. Thanks to Paul Poppen, PhD, for his expert assistance in planning and executing the statistical analyses. Andrew Nicholson, MD, and Mark Sklar, MD, guided our initial research on diabetes, and Larry Kushi, PhD, provided thoughtful advice along the way. John A. McDougall, MD, and Mary McDougall provided educational materials and wonderful recipes. Jennie Brand-Miller, PhD, of the University of Sydney, kindly answered many questions about her studies of the glycemic index and its use in clinical practice.

Stanley Talpers, MD, kept a watchful eye on medical issues for our participants, and Brad Moore, MD, served as our safety officer.

Special thanks to Ernest P. Noble, MD, PhD, and Terry Ritchie, PhD, of the University of California, Los Angeles, for their generosity and expertise in genetic analyses. Thank you to Donald S. Karcher, MD; Terry Costa; Luce Merino; Estela Day; Patrice Moore; and everyone at George Washington University clinical laboratory client services.

Cael Croft provided the wonderful medical illustrations in this book.

Finally, thank you to my literary agent, Brian DeFiore, and my editor, Marisa Vigilante, for helping to shape this book into its current form; and Bryanna Clark Grogan for providing wonderful recipes.

A New Approach to Diabetes

This book presents a revolutionary method for preventing, controlling, and reversing diabetes based on important research findings that have dramatically changed our understanding of this condition. When this book first appeared, the idea that diabetes could improve dramatically and sometimes even go away for all intents and purposes was a novel concept. The prevailing notion was "once you have diabetes, you'll always have diabetes," and the condition just seemed to lead to more and more complications. We have changed that scenario.

In studies by my research team, funded by the US government's National Institutes of Health and the Diabetes Action Research and Education Foundation, along with the work of other researchers, we have completely redesigned the dietary approach to diabetes. If your experience with diabetes has been one of gradually escalating medication doses, ever-increasing weight, and increasing worry about the risk of complications, you will learn how to reverse those trends.

We will focus on changes in your menu, not on drugs. Yes, medications often have their role. But I would much rather help you scale back on drugs—or eliminate them entirely. Doing that means rethinking the foods that you eat. Let me emphasize that you will not need to cut calories, limit carbohydrates, or stick to small portions. In fact, you can eat until you are full. If you get hungry between meals, you are free to eat more. What we will zero in on is the *type* of food you eat. That has emerged as the critical factor, as you will soon see.

A NEW IDEA

My father, Donald M. Barnard, MD, spent his entire life treating diabetes. He grew up on a family farm in the Midwest but soon realized that the cattle business was not for him. He decided to go to medical school, and after training at Boston's famed Joslin Clinic, he began work at a busy community hospital. He became known as the diabetes expert for the surrounding area. But he and the other doctors—and their patients—often found diabetes puzzling and frustrating. He recounted a telling comment made by the clinic's founder, Elliott P. Joslin, MD, about diabetes research: "Gentlemen, we don't need a big research grant. What we need is a new idea."

Dr. Joslin made that observation back in the 1950s, and the need has only grown more urgent as the incidence of the disease has exploded. Worldwide, more than 400 million people are living with diabetes. Until now, most have found the condition to be at best an exercise in drudgery. With daily blood tests and a growing list of medications that aim only to slow the disease's inevitable damage, a patient's life becomes a waiting game, with one complication arising after another—from nerve symptoms to visual changes and heart and kidney problems.

Now, at last, we have a much more powerful approach. I'm talking not just about a bold new idea, but about an entirely new approach to diabetes that has been tested and proven.

In a series of research studies conducted first with Georgetown University and George Washington University in Washington, DC, our research team has proven that many people with diabetes can think beyond delaying inevitable decline and improve their health dramatically. They can cut their blood sugar, increase insulin sensitivity, and reduce or eliminate medications, and they can do this with a simple set of diet changes. Unlike with medication treatments, the "side effects" of the menu change are good ones: weight loss, lower cholesterol levels, lower blood pressure, and increased energy.

From the beginning, our studies aimed higher and took a more aggressive approach to diabetes than clinicians had in the past. The first study was small—just 13 patients—and it tested a program that relied entirely on changes in diet. There was no new drug, no magical supplement—not even an exercise program. But the results were amazing. Two-thirds of patients improved so much that they were able to reduce or eliminate their medications within 12 weeks. The study was published in *Preventive Medicine* in 1999.[1]

Then, in a second study, this one involving 59 patients with varying degrees of blood sugar control—some healthy, others prediabetic or diabetic—we studied *why* diet change works. It became clear that the diet shift actually caused a fundamental change in the body itself. In 14 weeks, the diet led to a 24 percent improvement in insulin sensitivity—that is, the body's ability to respond to insulin, the sugar-storing hormone that is dysfunctional in diabetes. Participants whose blood sugar levels were in the abnormal range saw them promptly return to where they belonged. While exercise could increase the benefits even further, *diet changes alone* were powerful enough to boost insulin sensitivity and bring blood sugar under better control. The results were presented at the American Diabetes Association Scientific Meeting in 2004 and were published in the *American Journal of Medicine* in 2005.[2]

These studies suggested that this new approach may be the most powerful nutritional plan ever devised for diabetes. We can do more than try to *compensate* for malfunctioning insulin, as doctors have done for decades with various medications. Rather, we can help the body's own insulin work properly again by directly addressing—and improving—the cells' sensitivity to it, which is the key issue in type 2 diabetes. Even when the disease has evolved to the point of serious complications, it is not too late for marked improvements to occur.

Starting in 2003, with the support of the National Institutes of Health, we conducted a new research trial to compare our diet, head-to-head, against the guidelines promulgated by the American Diabetes Association at that time. These conventional guidelines seemed sensible and were well accepted. Millions of people followed them, carefully cutting calories and limiting carbohydrates. But all too often, a familiar story ensued: Despite everyone's best efforts, the disease typically worsened over time. Our goal was to see if we could improve things. The study was conducted with George Washington

University and the University of Toronto and included 99 individuals with type 2 diabetes. The participants were randomly assigned to either a standard diabetic diet based on the 2003 ADA guidelines or to the more aggressive diet you will learn about shortly. Along the way, I presented the study's initial results at scientific meetings of the ADA, the American Association of Diabetes Educators, and the American Public Health Association.

In a careful analysis that kept exercise and medication use constant, we found that the new diet controlled blood sugar three times more effectively than the previous "best" diet. It also accelerates weight loss and controlled cholesterol better than the old gold standard. Other investigators have showed that this kind of diet also has dramatic benefits for the heart and leads to a big improvement in blood pressure. It allows many individuals to take charge of their lives again and to return to health and vigor.

We then ran two studies with GEICO, the insurance company, to see how it would apply in the work setting in 10 different cities. In a word, it works great and is easy to implement. We have also documented its efficacy against more advanced diabetes, focusing on improvements in nerve symptoms.

This book translates these scientific breakthroughs into tools that you can use, including an easy-to-follow plan with simple diet guidelines.

A NEW UNDERSTANDING OF TYPE 1 DIABETES

Type 1 diabetes is much less common than type 2. It is usually diagnosed in childhood and is invariably treated with insulin—hence its former names, childhood-onset diabetes and insulin-dependent-diabetes.

Unlike people with type 2 diabetes, those with type 1 always need to take insulin. But they can use diet and lifestyle changes to keep doses to a minimum and reduce the risk of complications. We also have a new understanding of the *fundamental causes* of type 1 diabetes. It may surprise you to learn that the process that leads to type 1 diabetes begins when the body's immune system attacks the insulin-producing cells of the pancreas. As you will see, new research has revealed what appears to spark this attack and what can help to prevent it.

PERSONAL SUCCESS

Let's take a look at the experiences of real people who followed the program described in this book.

Nancy

Nancy learned about our research study from an advertisement in the *Washington Post*. She had been diagnosed with type 2 diabetes 8 years earlier. A cousin of hers had lost some of his eyesight to the disease, and failed kidneys left him on dialysis. Nancy did not want that to be her future. She was going to fight back.

Before she joined our study, things had been going in the wrong direction. Although she had followed a diet designed for diabetes, her blood sugar was gradually worsening, and the diet did nothing to stop her weight from creeping upward.

Two years after her diagnosis, her doctor put her on her first diabetes medication. Eventually, her doctor felt she needed two medications. Still her blood glucose level continued to rise. As she entered our study, her hemoglobin A1C level—the key index of blood glucose control, which ought to be below 7.0 percent—was an unhealthy 8.3 percent.

Nancy joined the study because she liked the focus on food rather than on drugs. With the explosion of diabetes in the population, she intuitively felt that the problem had to be the kinds of food we eat and that the solution had to be there, too.

We showed her how to change her diet. There were no limits on how much she could eat or on how many calories or grams of carbohydrates she could have. But we did ask her to make a major change in the *type* of food she chose.

At first, we also asked her *not* to exercise—that is, not to change her exercise habits—because we wanted to see what diet changes alone could do. That suited her just fine—she was very busy at her office, working long hours every day, and exercise was not exactly her thing. At least not yet.

As she began to follow our recommendations, her weight started to fall, along with her blood glucose, the latter with surprising speed. After years of going up and up and up, the trend started to reverse. After 11 weeks, she stood on the scale: She had lost 14 pounds. And when she rolled up her sleeve and we checked her A1C, we found that it had dropped from 8.3 percent to 6.9 percent. All in about 3 months' time. Her insulin sensitivity was returning.

Nancy's blood sugar continued to fall. In fact, it fell so much that it became clear that her medications were now too strong for her. The combination of the drugs she had been taking, along with the new, powerful diet changes, actually left her blood sugar too low. It was time to reduce her medications. But as we cut back on her doses, it turned out not to be enough. After several more months, we had to stop one of them altogether.

A little more than a year after joining the study, she was 40 pounds lighter. She stopped her diabetes medications, and yet her A1C is better than it was before—6.8 percent at her last test.

"The payoff is just incredible," she said. "But it's not just the weight loss. My numbers have gotten dramatically better."

And there was more—another benefit she had not anticipated. For years, she had had arthritis pain so severe she could not open a jar. After a few months of a new diet, she suddenly realized that her arthritis symptoms were completely gone. (There is actually a fascinating body of scientific literature on diet and arthritis, which I summarized in an earlier book, *Foods That Fight Pain.*) The best part of the story: Nancy's experience is not unusual for people who make the diet changes you will read about shortly.

Vance

Vance was just 31 years old when he was diagnosed with diabetes. He had just changed to a new doctor, and the diagnosis came after a routine blood test. Both of his mother's parents had had the disease, but up until that point, Vance had been in more or less good health. He had been a police officer for 12 years and now worked in a bank, and he was not in the habit of calling in sick.

Diabetes changed everything. "If I didn't lose a leg or go blind, I could end up on dialysis," he said. And the truth was, he was not in such perfect shape. He had gradually gained weight over the years, and at just under 6 feet tall, he weighed 276 pounds. "I didn't really take my diet or my health very seriously," he said. "I grew up on steak sandwiches, pork chops, and chicken. We had barbecues and cookouts. We had some vegetables, but not a lot of fresh foods. I didn't exercise. I just didn't take any of this very seriously."

Along with weight problems came difficulties with sexual performance. Impotence affects many men with diabetes and is common in men who are overweight. His doctor started him on metformin, a commonly prescribed medication for reducing blood sugar.

Vance learned about our research study and decided to volunteer—despite a few misgivings about the prospect of changing his diet. "I never had any diet restrictions or rules before," he said. "I never tried to control my diet before. I always ate whatever I wanted." But his wife had been a vegetarian for some time, and she was excited that Vance was ready for a change, too.

The payoff came pretty quickly. His weight started to fall, and over a year's time, he lost—to his surprise—about 60 pounds. His A1C, which had been 9.5 percent at the beginning of the study, fell to 7.1 percent after just 2 months. Fourteen months into the study, it had dropped to 5.3 percent. His doctor was thrilled and said it was time to stop the metformin.

One more surprise: His problems with sexual performance virtually disappeared within 3 months. "I haven't been in this good shape since I was in the police academy. It is like a weight has been lifted off of me," he said. "When I told my mother what I was doing—that I had changed my diet—she was so happy, she nearly cried, because my dad died at 30. When my grandfather died, I was the oldest male in my immediate family. We tend to check out pretty quick. But she saw I was on a different path. I was taking care of myself."

SUCCESS

As soon as the first edition of this book appeared, we began to hear from many more people who were putting this method to use and achieving surprising results. A reader in England sent this message:

> I was diagnosed with type 2 last September and was given the standard diet/lifestyle advice by my doctor and his colleagues here in the UK. Initially my diabetes was mild and was managed simply with diet/exercise. With time, however, there was deterioration, requiring stronger and stronger medication, and I began to experience the early stages of typical diabetes complications. I was given a copy of Neal's book by a caring and concerned friend. I was skeptical at first because all the (difficult to maintain) diet changes I had made to that point did not seem to be of any use in tackling the problem. However, I embraced the plan in the book and really began to enjoy eating the foods recommended.
>
> Three months after starting out on Neal's diet, I have had my second (since diagnosis) review. I was called into the doctor's office at very short notice with no explanation given by the administrator on the phone, just being told that "we need to see you today to discuss your blood results from last week." Obviously I was anxious, to say the least, and was quite worried just what bad news the doc was going to deliver. The doctor called me in however to ask me what I was doing because "your blood picture is now more normal than mine, and I don't have diabetes." He then said "I can't tell you that you no longer have diabetes because there is no cure for diabetes, but technically, you don't."
>
> My doctor was shocked at my blood numbers; he said that the most improvement he has ever seen up to that point was typically no more than 5 to 10 percent in his best-managed diabetes patients. My blood numbers were apparently more than 60 percent better than my last set of results in January

(before I started Neal's diet). My doctor is now recommending Neal's diet to his other patients with diabetes.

Another reader, Patricia, was working as a defense analyst at the
Pentagon. For most of her life, she had struggled with her weight, and
eventually she was 95 pounds heavier than she wanted to be. At age 58,
she developed diabetes and had blocked arteries in her heart. She was
making trips to doctors' offices much more often than she would have
liked and was taking 13 pills and two shots a day.

But she learned about our approach and put it to work. Patricia
ended up *losing* 95 pounds. She got off all her diabetes medications. She
has more energy than she has had in years. Her husband followed her
lead, and he slimmed down, too. They are doing things they couldn't
do before, and they feel great.

A woman in Portland wrote that she had started gaining weight after
the birth of her second child. She worked evenings at a catalog call
center, and when she got off work, she found herself at the drive-thru
on the way home, ordering unhealthy things and more food than she
needed. Over time, she gained almost 100 pounds.

That extra weight took a real toll, and it gradually robbed her of
things she loved to do. One year, her family went to Disneyland, and
she found that she was really not able to walk around the various sights.
She had no energy, and her feet hurt. After a half-hour, she was pooped,
and she had to leave.

One day, the occupational nurse at work called her urgently to let
her know the results of some blood tests she had had. Her fasting blood
sugar was 278, which looked like out-of-control diabetes.

This was a major wake-up call. She was not just heavy; she was in
trouble.

Well, she found information from my team about tackling weight
problems and diabetes. Our method focused on food and allowed her
to eat as much as she wanted, zeroing in on the *type* of food she ate.
That sounded really appealing, and she jumped in.

In the first 3 weeks, she lost 7 pounds, and her blood sugar was starting to fall, too. After a year, she was down 60 pounds. And today she is
at the weight she wants to be.

And what about her diabetes? Well, her A1C blood test was 10.1 when she started—that's way into the diabetic range. But it gradually came down and down and down, and today it is well *below* the diabetic range. And her cholesterol plummeted 63 points.

And her energy is back. Remember the problems she had trying to walk around Disneyland? Well, today she is on her feet for hours at a time, running training courses for new employees. And she has energy to burn.

Her skin used to be blotchy and red. And now it's back to the way it should be. Headaches, stomachaches, and pains in her feet have all gone away, and she feels great.

She has taken control, shedding that weight and getting her energy back. And she loves eating healthful foods that work for her, not against her.

There are many, many more stories of great success from real people. But now is the time for you to begin your own success story.

TAKING CONTROL

The diet embraced by Nancy, Vance, and the others you have read about here—and that I hope you are about to begin—is designed to do much more than simply palliate diabetes, as other diets do. It is designed to tackle the fundamental causes of the disease.

As those who participated in our study learned, blood sugar levels that creep steadily upward can also fall. The road to diabetes is in fact a two-way street.

Whether you have type 2 diabetes and want to gain control of your health or have type 1 diabetes and need to reduce the disease's intrusion on your life, this program was designed with you in mind.

However, our research—and this book—also targets a broader purpose. More and more people, including a surprising number of children, are diagnosed with diabetes every day. They and their families pay a high personal price with the condition. And clinics, health maintenance organizations, insurers, and government programs are struggling to keep up with prescription costs, doctor visits, and hospitalization charges for its many complications. For many people at risk, it is simply a matter of time before they are diagnosed. It is our hope that a new direction in diet and nutrition, if applied broadly enough, can go a long way toward solving these problems.

This program is truly a revolution in the way we think about this otherwise unforgiving disease. Diabetes is no longer a condition you simply have to live with. It need not slowly and inevitably get worse. Quite the opposite. If you have diabetes, it is time for you to get your life back.

We will not cater to your diabetes. Rather, this program is designed to help you understand the *cause* of diabetes and how to *correct it* to the fullest extent that diet and lifestyle changes possibly can. If you do not have the disease but are at risk, this is a powerful program for preventing it.

"Is this program for me?" you may be asking. The answer is an emphatic yes. Here's why.

- **Whether you like to cook or prefer to eat at restaurants, you can easily make the diet changes you need.** I make this point because some people imagine that changing their diet means making every meal in their own kitchens. Translation: hours and hours of work. If you inwardly groan at that thought, I certainly sympathize: I learned long ago that my temperament is not suited to spending much time in the kitchen. Perhaps I was born with the "room service gene," and maybe you were, too. So I will show you how to plan a healthful menu and how to make it work for you whether or not you like to cook. Many of our research participants travel, eat at restaurants, or eat in their company cafeterias. This program worked for them, and it can work for you.

- **It does not matter whether you love exercise or have never been able to stick with an exercise plan.** The improvements described above were made *without exercise.* In fact, our research studies typically omit exercise because we need to isolate the effect of diet changes in order to put them to a good test. Having said that, exercise is an important part of any diabetes treatment regimen, and this book will show you how to bring it into your life in a sensible, safe, and effective way. If, however, you are unable to engage in significant exercise because of joint problems, a heart condition, or severe obesity, or if you find you're just not able to stick with an exercise program, you will be glad to know that the benefits of our diet change are not dependent on any alteration of your activity levels.

• **If you have felt that you just cannot stick with a diet, I completely understand.** That's why we will focus solely on what you eat, not *how much*. You can eat until you are full and have snacks when you want them. You will have to invest some energy, however: You will have to learn to think about food in new ways. And you will have to unlearn some old, outdated notions. And if you have been overweight, it is very likely that you will have to buy some new clothes!

WHAT DOES IT MEAN TO *REVERSE* DIABETES?

Most people with diabetes find themselves on a road leading toward gradually increasing weight, slowly rising blood sugar, higher doses of medications, and worsening complications. Reversing diabetes means reversing this trend. If weight is an issue, it can come down—gradually, but decisively. Blood glucose values that have gone up can also come down. Doses of medications that have risen again and again can come down, too. Symptoms such as neuropathy—nerve pain in the feet and legs—can improve and even disappear. Heart disease can be reversed.

Will the disease go away completely? Some people would argue that once someone has diabetes, that person will always have it, even if blood tests improve so much that the condition is no longer diagnosable. What they mean is that the genetic traits that made type 2 diabetes possible do not go away, and type 1 diabetes requires continued insulin treatments regardless of how well you adjust your diet.

It is not possible to say in advance how far you can go. Will you be able to reduce your medication doses, eliminate some or perhaps all of your medications, or drive your blood sugar down so far that no one would ever know you once had diabetes? These are questions your own experience will answer, but I can promise this book will teach you what you need to know about putting a powerful food prescription to work. The rest of the story is yours to write.

I would be very grateful if you would let others know what you are doing and perhaps lend this book to your friends or family members who have diabetes. We know that we can turn this disease around for individuals, but conquering an international epidemic is a tall order, and it requires a team effort. I hope you will join in this important cause along with health professionals, research participants, and their families.

Thank you, and the very best of luck with this program.

PART 1

The Breakthrough

CHAPTER 1

The New Basics

In recent years, much of what we thought we knew about diabetes has been turned on its head. What is now coming into focus is an understanding of its fundamental *causes*, and that gives us power we never had before.

To make sure we are at the same starting point, let me walk you through the basics: symptoms, diabetes types, and typical treatments as they are currently used. Then I will show you what's new.

HOW DO WE KNOW IT'S DIABETES?

First, let's make sense of the symptoms. Diabetes may arrive with no symptoms at all, but often it starts with fatigue. For no apparent reason, your spark is just no longer there. It may also seem that you are losing water more rapidly than you should be, which is to say that you make trips to the bathroom more often than usual. And you are thirsty: You find yourself drinking a surprising amount of water.

Here is what is going on: The fundamental problem is that sugar is not able to pass from your bloodstream into the cells of your body. From that single problem come a great many others, like one domino knocking over another and another and another.

The sugar we are speaking of is glucose—one of the smallest and simplest sugar molecules. In this case, *sugar* is not just another word for junk food or empty calories. The fact is that the cells of your body use this kind of sugar—glucose—as an energy source. Like gasoline for your car or jet fuel for an airplane, glucose is your body's fuel. It powers your movements, your thoughts, and more or less everything you do.

And that is exactly the problem. If glucose is unable to enter your cells, they are deprived of their basic fuel, so you lose your energy. That is why you are fatigued. If your muscles do not have the glucose they need for power, you tire easily.

Meanwhile, the glucose that cannot get into your muscle cells builds up in your bloodstream. It becomes more and more concentrated in the blood, and eventually it starts to pass through the kidneys and ends up in your urine.*

Now, as glucose passes through your kidneys, it carries water along with it—lots of water, hence all those trips to the bathroom. What follows, naturally, is thirst—you are losing all those fluids. So fatigue, frequent urination, and thirst are all symptoms of one problem: Glucose is having trouble getting into your cells.

You may also find that you are losing weight. And no, this is not an especially welcome event—not in this situation. You lose weight because your cells are in essence starving. Nutrients cannot enter your cells, so your body is malnourished. Yes, even if you are eating plenty of food, nutrients and fuel are unable to get where they are needed.

Every day, people arrive at doctors' offices complaining of fatigue, frequent urination, thirst, and sometimes unexplained weight loss. The doctor takes a blood sample, finds an unusually high level of glucose in the blood, and diagnoses diabetes. The doctor then advises the patient that it is essential to get blood sugar under control. An overly large amount of glucose flooding through the bloodstream day after day can harm the arteries. Left unchecked, it can damage the heart and the delicate blood vessels of the eyes, kidneys, and extremities.

But as we have shown in our research studies, the road to high

---

* The passage of glucose from the bloodstream into the urine led to the technical name doctors use for diabetes: diabetes mellitus. *Diabetes* comes from a Greek word meaning "to pass through," and *mellitus* is the Latin word for "honey" or "sweet."

How Doctors Diagnose Diabetes

Doctors diagnose diabetes if:

- Your blood glucose level is 126 mg/dl (7.0 mmol/l)* or higher after an 8-hour fast.

- Your blood glucose is 200 mg/dl (11.1 mmol/l) or higher after a 2-hour glucose tolerance test. This is a test in which you drink a syrup containing 75 grams of glucose, and your blood glucose value is measured.

- Your A1C blood test is 6.5 percent or higher. A1C is a test that reflects your blood sugar control over the preceding 3 months or so, unlike a blood glucose test, which will tend to rise and fall from minute to minute under the influence of foods, physical activity, medications, stress, and other factors. What the A1C test actually measures is how much glucose has entered your red blood cells and become stuck to hemoglobin. If you have had a lot of glucose in your blood, a fair amount of it gets into your cells and sticks to your hemoglobin.

*US medical laboratories measure glucose in milligrams per deciliter (mg/dl). In most other countries, glucose is measured in millimoles per liter (mmol/l). As you will see, the same units are used in cholesterol measurements.

blood sugar is a two-way street. When you change your diet and make other healthful improvements, a rising glucose level can fall. Sometimes the change can be so dramatic that no doctor looking at you afterward would ever guess that you had once been diagnosed with diabetes.

Diabetes Types

A diagnosis of diabetes—or prediabetes—means the insulin in your body is not doing its job adequately. Insulin is a hormone that moves sugar from your bloodstream into the cells of your body, among other functions. It acts like a key, opening a door to the cell, so to speak, and allowing nutrients inside. When insulin arrives at the cell's surface and opens the door, glucose is able to enter the cell, which uses it for power.

If for some reason your body is not making insulin, the result is rising blood glucose levels. Similarly, your blood glucose rises if your cells resist insulin's actions—the key goes in the lock, but the door will not open.

Diabetes comes in three main types, called type 1, type 2, and gestational diabetes, plus some variants you may need to know about. Let's look at each one.

Type 1 diabetes usually manifests in childhood or young adulthood. It used to be called childhood-onset or insulin-dependent diabetes. In type 1 diabetes, something has damaged the pancreas's ability to produce insulin, and you need to get it from an outside source—typically by injection. However, research has revealed a great deal about how diet changes can reduce the risk that diabetes will bring any serious complications your way, as you will see in Chapter 3.

In addition, we know more than ever about the causes of the disease, arming us with more power to prevent it. The damage to the insulin-producing cells is caused by the biological equivalent of "friendly fire." That is, it is caused by the body's immune system—our white blood cells that are supposed to fight bacteria and viruses. These cells ought to protect you, but instead they have attacked the cells of the pancreas, destroying its ability to produce insulin. In Chapter 3, we will look at what triggers this process. It may surprise you to learn that foods—particularly the foods infants are fed within the first months of life—are leading suspects.

When type 1 diabetes manifests in people who are beyond early adulthood, the term *latent autoimmune diabetes of adults* (LADA) is sometimes used. But the disease is still type 1 diabetes.

Type 2 diabetes used to be called adult-onset diabetes, or sometimes non–insulin-dependent diabetes. About 9 out of 10 people with diabetes have type 2. Most people with this form of the disease still produce insulin; the problem is that their cells resist it. Insulin tries to bring glucose into the cells, but the cells respond like a door with a malfunctioning lock. In response to these sluggish cells, your body produces more and more insulin, trying to overcome the resistance. If the body's insulin supply cannot overcome the resistance, glucose simply builds up in your blood.

Diabetes drugs work to counteract this problem: Some make your

Insulin Is Made in the Pancreas

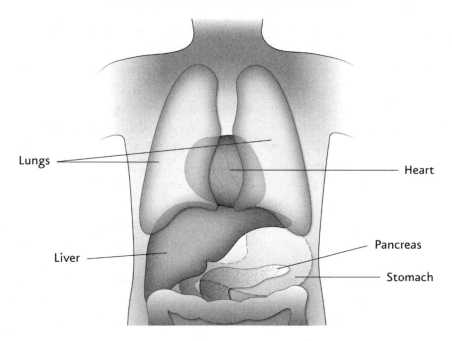

Lungs —

Heart —

Liver —

Pancreas —

Stomach —

Insulin is made in the pancreas, an organ located just behind your stomach that is about the size and shape of a TV remote control. In fact, remote control is what the pancreas is all about. It sends insulin into the bloodstream to travel to the cells of your body to help them take in glucose from the bloodstream. In type 1 diabetes, the pancreas has stopped making insulin. In type 2 and gestational diabetes, the pancreas is usually able to make insulin, but the body's cells resist its action.

cells more responsive to insulin. Others cause your pancreas to release more insulin into the bloodstream or block your liver from sending extra glucose into the blood.

Until now, most diabetes diets have tried to compensate for the cells' resistance to insulin's action, too. They limited the amount of sugar in your diet. They have also limited starch (complex carbohydrate) because starch is actually made from many glucose molecules joined together in a chain. During digestion, starch breaks down to release natural sugars into the blood. The idea is that if you do not get too much carbohydrate at any one time, your cells will not be over-whelmed with too much glucose. For people on medications, typical diet plans have aimed to keep the amount of sugar or starch fairly constant from meal to meal and from day to day so the amount of medication required to help your body process glucose—your daily dosage—can stay the same, too. In short, these diets have guided you on what, when, and how much to eat.

New research has changed everything, however. We can now use diet changes to influence insulin sensitivity directly. So, as you will see shortly, the nutrition prescription has been completely rewritten to take advantage of this new understanding.

Gestational diabetes is similar to type 2 except that it occurs during pregnancy. While it typically disappears after childbirth, it is a sign of insulin resistance, and that means that type 2 diabetes may be around the corner. With the same sorts of steps that tackle type 2 diabetes, we can often stop gestational diabetes from ever turning into type 2.

Maturity Onset Diabetes of the Young (MODY). Rarely, a genetic characteristic can cause the pancreas to produce insufficient insulin. The gene is typically dominant. The affected individual is very likely to develop high blood sugars, even though he or she may not be overweight or have insulin-resistant cells. Because the pancreas contin-ues to produce some insulin, insulin injections may not be needed. The treatment is similar to type 2.

Prediabetes is the term used when your blood glucose level is higher than normal, but not high enough for a diagnosis of diabetes. For most people, it means that you have insulin resistance and are on your way to developing type 2 diabetes, unless you take steps now to improve your health, especially through changes in your eating habits. This term applies when:

- Your fasting blood glucose level is between 100 and 125 mg/dl (between 5.6 and 6.9 mmol/l).

- Your blood glucose is between 140 and 199 mg/dl (between 7.8 and 11.1 mmol/l) after a 2-hour glucose tolerance test.

- Your A1C blood test is between 5.7 and 6.4 percent.

The good news is that the same steps that help people tackle type 2 diabetes are also effective for helping people with prediabetes to improve, often decisively.

GENES ARE NOT DESTINY

Diabetes runs in families, but don't take that to mean that if one of your parents has diabetes, a similar diagnosis has to be your fate as well. You can change things.

Let's take a look at type 1 diabetes first. Many children are born with genes that make it possible for them to develop type 1 diabetes, but most of them never do. In fact, even among identical twins, when one twin has type 1 diabetes, the other has less than a 40 percent chance of having it.[1] What makes the difference, apparently, is the environment, particularly the foods the child is exposed to early in life (e.g., cow's milk); viral infections; and perhaps other factors.

Genes play a similar role in type 2 diabetes. Many years before diabetes ever manifests, special tests can detect insulin resistance in young adults who have inherited a tendency toward type 2 diabetes from their parents. If they eat the same kinds of foods their parents did, they are very likely headed for a diagnosis. Abundant evidence shows, however, that changes in diet and lifestyle can cut the odds that diabetes will occur. When it does occur, diet can dramatically alter its course.

The point is this: Some genes are dictators, and others are not. The genes for hair color or eye color, for example, really are dictators. If they call for you to have brown hair or blue eyes, you can't argue. But the genes for diabetes are more like committees. They do not give orders; they make suggestions.

If our genes call for diabetes, we do not necessarily have to listen to them. We have more control than you might imagine.

EATING PATTERNS FOR DIABETES

If you have diabetes, chances are you were given printed guidelines on what to eat and what to avoid. Perhaps you have met with a dietitian, and you may have been referred to a diabetes class. If you are like many people, you may have found your diet tough to sustain.

For many years, diets for people with diabetes were designed to provide basic nutrition while also keeping calorie intake and food choices reasonably stable over the course of the day and from one day to the next, as you saw above. The idea was that if you had no carbohydrates for breakfast but then had a big carb-fest later in the day, your blood sugar would change erratically. Similarly, if you had lots of starchy foods on Monday but went low-carb the rest of the week, your blood sugar would be all over the map, and your medications could not keep up with you.

That approach sounds logical, but it was devised before the causes of insulin resistance were known and has turned out to be of limited value. Many people have trouble sticking with it. Now that we understand more about what is happening inside your cells to cause diabetes, we can choose foods more strategically. That means diet changes that are simpler and more effective, as you will see in the following chapters.

The American Diabetes Association now gives a thumbs-up to several different eating patterns, including vegetarian and vegan diets, the semi-vegetarian "DASH diet," low-fat diets, low-carbohydrate diets, and "Mediterranean diets." However, we now have good scientific evidence that allows us to see which diet changes really work best over the long run, and soon you will be putting that power to work.

DRUGS AND MONEY

The diet changes you will read about in this book are powerful. Unfortunately, the power of nutrition is neglected in many medical practices, and in the process, diabetes treatment is reduced to a series of prescriptions.

Don't misunderstand me. Diabetes medications can be lifesaving. They can reduce your blood sugar and, over the long run, cut your risk of complications. And if diet and lifestyle changes do not do the job, it can be a serious mistake to forgo medications. But some doctors and patients view medications as the only tools at their disposal. The marketing of pharmaceuticals has so dominated medical practice that many doctors give little more than lip service to diet and exercise, which can often be dramatically effective.

Open any diabetes journal and you will see expensive advertisements for this drug and that drug.

If you were to leaf through the mail that floods doctors' offices, you would see information about medical courses, symposia, and online educational programs, all paid for by drug companies trumpeting their products. These companies cater full dinners to lure doctors to presentations about one or another application of their drugs. While many doctors find such events distasteful, they are required to attend medical courses to maintain their hospital or university affiliations, and drug companies have cornered the medical education market.

At the ADA annual meeting, drug company representatives arrive at the loading dock looking as if they are preparing to put on an enormous political convention. They erect huge display booths costing hundreds of thousands of dollars staffed with armies of sales personnel ready to provide gifts, food, musical entertainment, and trinkets of all kinds, all designed to woo the clinicians in attendance.

And, of course, drug companies target consumers directly. Turn on a television in any American city, and you will soon be inundated by commercials asking you to speak with your doctor about all manner of medications. They make diabetes sound almost like fun, and their latest products add to your modern lifestyle.

You, the drug consumer, are stuck with the bill for all this. A typical diabetes pill contains a few cents' worth of active medication, but the retail cost is heavily inflated by its manufacturer's promotional expenses and its continued efforts to find yet another pill that can carve out more of the market share.

The diabetes business is not limited to drugs. Patients need to buy glucose testing equipment, too. While glucose meters are not terribly expensive, manufacturers charge a small fortune for the supplies that go with them, much like the shaving-product companies that give away free razors to sell expensive blades. The test strips that fit into a typical glucose meter cost about $1 each, and a person might use anywhere from one to eight strips per day. Add up the costs of doctor visits, laboratory tests, medication, and glucose monitoring equipment, and diabetes becomes a phenomenally expensive disease.

It is my hope that as the power of nutritional changes is more fully appreciated, the commercial aspects of diabetes will take a backseat. The US government has already invested in research on diet and diabetes, and that investment will continue to pay important dividends. We must also turn our attention to putting what we have learned about nutrition to work. That means encouraging doctors to focus on diet first, pushing insurers to cover dietetic counseling for patients and their families, educating parents about nutritional approaches to help prevent type 1 diabetes in their children, and working with schools to serve healthful meals so children are not sent down the road to overweight and diabetes, as a great many currently are. These measures could control the so-called diseases of affluence far more effectively than doctors are able to at present, dramatically reducing the need for medications in the first place.

Each person with diabetes has a unique ability to heal and return to health. This ability differs from one person to the next, but in our studies, we have not seen age, weight, or any other factor to be a barrier to improvement.

The remainder of this book will show you what I believe to be the most powerful dietary approach to diabetes that is currently known.

CHAPTER 2

Reversing Type 2 Diabetes

Remarkably, my research has shown that it is possible to reverse diabetes—to decrease blood sugar, medication doses, and the risk of complications—and this chapter will show you how, using surprisingly simple diet changes. I will also share some surprising new findings about the causes of type 2 diabetes—changes inside your body's cells that can be detected years before diabetes starts. Evidence suggests that switching to a healthier diet has a powerful influence on the workings of your cells, as you will see.

All doctors and dietitians recognize that if you have diabetes, your body does not process sugar very well, which is to say that the amount of sugar in your bloodstream is too high. Researchers learned long ago that if it stays high, you are at risk for many health problems down the road.

To lower your blood sugar, most medical professionals are likely to prescribe a diet that includes very little sugar. They will also ask you to limit starchy foods—such as bread, potatoes, rice, and pasta—because in your digestive tract, starch breaks apart to release sugar (that is, glucose). It seems to make sense—if your body cannot handle sugar, you have to be careful about eating too much sugar and anything that turns into it. Your medical team will also encourage you to space out your intake of starches and sugars throughout the day—and from one day to the next—so that it stays fairly even over time. Diabetes diets also generally cut calories to help you lose weight and limit certain fats to reduce the risk of heart disease and other complications. That, in a nutshell, is a typical "traditional" diabetes diet.

It is certainly logical, and some people greatly benefit from following it. The problem is that for most people, this sort of diet change has only a very limited effect. Weight loss is usually modest, and the diet alone typically is not enough to bring blood sugar under control.

Sooner or later, you and your doctor are likely to decide that the "diabetes diet" is not helping very much, and your doctor will add various drugs. You may need one, two, or even three different oral medications. Eventually, your doctor may consider adding insulin injections. And because many people with diabetes also have high blood pressure or high cholesterol levels, doctors often add medications to tackle these problems, too. Instead of helping you reduce or avoid medications, the diet seems to be a stepping-stone on the way to an ever-increasing list of drugs.

The first glimmer that there might be a better way came from a look at the prevalence of diabetes around the world. Large population studies showed that diabetes was rare in Japan, China, Thailand, and other Asian countries. It was similarly rare in parts of Africa.

These studies also showed something else: People in countries where diabetes was uncommon were not following anything like a "diabetes diet." They did not avoid carbohydrates; they ate starchy foods every day. In Asia and Africa, rice and other grains, starchy vegetables, bean dishes, and noodles are staples. In fact, researchers found that people in these countries ate considerably more carbohydrates than North Americans or Europeans do, yet diabetes was relatively rare. So were weight problems. While obesity is found in more than 30 percent of American adults, it occurred in less than 1 percent of Japanese adults following a traditional diet. Heart disease and several forms of cancer were rare, too. Longevity among Japanese adults was better than that of North Americans or Europeans.

That is, until they moved to Vancouver—or Seattle, Chicago, Atlanta, or Washington, DC. For a Japanese adult, a move to North

America dramatically increased the risk of diabetes. Heart disease, obesity, and other problems became much more common, too.

Now, if you are worrying that I am going to ask you to adopt a traditional Japanese diet, relax. That's not a bad idea, but it is not what this book is about. I raise this international comparison simply to make an important point: *Carbohydrates do not cause diabetes.* And a diet that focuses on keeping carbohydrates out of your diet is not a powerful way to manage—let alone reverse—the disease. If anything, healthy complex carbohydrates help prevent it.

Think about what happens when an Asian man or woman switches to a Western lifestyle. Hamburgers, fried chicken, cheese, and other Western fare come into the diet, while rice and noodles are gradually forgotten. The diet becomes fattier and much higher in protein, while carbohydrate-rich rice and noodles and other starchy foods fall by the wayside.

Tragically, that is exactly what is happening. What's more, Asian men and women need not leave home for these changes to occur. McDonald's has come to them; Burger King, KFC, and other Western eating habits have also invaded Asia. Meat, cheese, and other greasy foods are displacing rice and vegetables.

As the Japanese diet has become Westernized, the prevalence of diabetes has exploded. In studies of adults in Japan over age 40, diabetes prevalence was between 1 and 5 percent prior to 1980. By 1990, it had gone up to 11 to 12 percent.[1] Statistical projections suggest it will rise even further. It turns out that the genes that allow diabetes to occur are surprisingly common among the Japanese, but as long as they stuck to their rice-based traditional diet, the disease was mostly held in check. The diabetes genes lay dormant, like seeds on dry soil. Once rice fell out of fashion and Western eating habits took hold, the genetic traits started to show themselves.

So, if people in Asia or Africa who eat lots of carbohydrates have very little diabetes, and if the disease becomes more and more common as carbohydrates are excluded from the diet, researchers have had to conclude that a high-carbohydrate diet is not the cause of the disease. In fact, the culprit seems to be lurking in our Western diets.

The inescapable fact is that the problem is not carbohydrates (that is, sugar and starch). *The problem is in how the body processes them.* If we can repair your body's ability to absorb and use carbohydrates, not only can you enjoy healthy carbohydrate-rich foods without worry, but diabetes itself ought to improve—perhaps even go away.

A look inside your body will show you what I mean.

A LOOK INSIDE YOUR BODY

Your pancreas, an organ in your abdomen, produces insulin. As you know by now, insulin is a hormone, and the pancreas sends it into your bloodstream to travel to the various cells of the body. Like a key sliding into a lock, insulin attaches to a receptor on the cell's surface and causes the cell membrane to permit glucose to enter. Insulin does the same thing for the next cell, and the next, and the next. It attaches to a receptor on the cell's surface, opens the door, and ushers glucose in.

In type 2 diabetes, this system does not work properly. Your pancreas makes insulin, and insulin travels to each cell, but when it arrives, it has trouble opening the door. It is as if the lock has somehow become jammed, and the key no longer works. This is insulin resistance. Yes, the insulin "key" is there, but it has trouble doing its job. Glucose cannot get into the cells, and it builds up in the bloodstream.

Imagine the workings of a lock on a typical door. What if someone were to jam chewing gum into the lock? There is nothing wrong with your key and really nothing wrong with the lock except that it is now filled with gum. To make it work again, we need to clean it out.

The new approach to diabetes is based on cleaning out your biological locks. Our goal is to help your insulin "key" work the way it is supposed to.

THE NEW DIABETES DIET

As far back as the early 1900s, researchers were adjusting people's diets to try to improve insulin sensitivity.[2, 3] Over the years, many—like me—have been inspired by the fact that foods that are commonly eaten in Asia or Africa somehow help prevent diabetes.

In 1979, researchers at the University of Kentucky studied 20 men with type 2 diabetes, all of whom had been taking an average of 26 units of insulin per day. The experimental diet included plenty of vegetables, fruits, whole grains, and beans, so it was high in fiber and carbohydrate. The diet was nearly vegetarian, with very little animal fat—in fact, very little fat of any kind.

After just 16 days on the program, more than half of the men were able to stop taking insulin entirely, and their blood sugar levels were *lower* than before.[4] For the remaining men, insulin doses were cut dramatically. That was an amazing and rapid result. But the study was short, and the participants lived on the research ward for its duration. It was unclear whether a similar result would be seen in people living on their own and preparing their own meals and whether it would be sustained over the long term.

A study conducted at the University of California, Los Angeles— 197 men enrolled in a 3-week diet change and exercise program— showed much the same thing. Of this group, 140 were able to discontinue their medications.[5] That was a great result, and it occurred very quickly. The study's limitation from our point of view was that it could not separate the effects of diet from those of exercise. Both are important, of course, but if we want to track down the best diet for diabetes, it is important to keep everything else constant while the diet is being tested.

Several years ago, my research team began a series of studies to see what diet alone could do. We tested a diet that focused not on limiting carbohydrates but rather on getting as much fat off the plate as possible. We thought if we could do that, perhaps we could clean out the "lock" mechanism that opens the cell doors.

We began with a small pilot study, which I mentioned briefly in the Introduction. Most of the participants were surprised to see rice, pasta, sweet potatoes, and beans on the menu and even more surprised that the diet did not limit carbohydrates at all. No matter how long they had had diabetes or how nervous they felt about the idea of putting carbohydrates back onto their plates, we put no limit on carbs at all.

There was also no limit on portions. Most of our participants were overweight, but even so, we did not ask them to limit portions or cut calories.

What we zeroed in on was fat. We aimed to clean all the grease out of the participants' diets. So, instead of bacon and eggs for breakfast, they had to choose from old-fashioned oatmeal, half a cantaloupe, or whole grain toast. If they had chili for lunch, it was veggie chili. Instead of pasta topped with meat sauce, they got meatless marinara. For the duration of the study, we asked them to set aside animal products completely and stick to vegetarian foods.

Needless to say, if there are no animal products in the diet, there is not a single drop of animal fat. We kept the use of vegetable oils as minimal as possible, too. And, in order to isolate the effects of the diet, we asked the participants not to alter their normal activity patterns; no one was to add exercise to the regimen. Now, exercise is an important part of any healthy lifestyle, and ordinarily we would strongly encourage it. But this was a test of the diet alone, and for scientific reasons, exercise was not to be part of it.

At the end of the study period, everyone weighed in. In just 12 weeks, the average participant had lost 16 pounds. Their fasting blood sugar had dropped 28 percent. Two-thirds of the participants on diabetes medications were able to reduce or discontinue them in that short period of time.[6] All this occurred without any limits on calories, portions, or carbohydrates and without exercise. These effects were significantly greater than those seen in a control group carefully following the diet guidelines of the American Diabetes Association (ADA).

That was impressive. But *why* did it happen? How does a diet that gives a green light to pasta, rice, and all the other foods that people with diabetes thought they had to live without—and one that completely disregards calories and avoids exercise—cause blood sugar to plummet and weight to easily drop away?

To answer that question, we designed another study. This one included a group of women who were moderately or severely overweight but did not have diabetes. Once again, we zeroed in on animal fat and vegetable oils. Our participants set animal products aside and kept oils to a bare minimum. And they were free to implement the diet guidelines in their own way, whether they ate at home or ate out, so it was a good test of how the diet would work in real life. For one person, eating out might have meant mushroom stroganoff with steamed vegetables; for another, it might have been vegetable sushi with miso soup and salad. As long as they avoided animal products and kept oils to a minimum, they were free to shape their meals to their liking.

For comparison, we included a control group whose members followed what you might think of as a typical cholesterol-lowering diet. It cut back on red meat while emphasizing poultry and fish along with plenty of vegetables, fruits, and whole grains.

The results were quick and impressive. The vegetarian group participants lost about a pound per week; after 14 weeks, they had lost an average of 13 pounds, compared to 8 pounds for the control group.[7]

By now, it was no surprise that this diet causes weight loss, but we went a step further. We sent our participants to the laboratory for a glucose tolerance test, which allowed us to measure how their bodies responded to sugar and how well their bodies' insulin was working. Each participant swallowed a dose of sugary syrup, and we took blood samples every half hour to measure rises in blood sugar and insulin. From these laboratory data, we were able to calculate each woman's insulin sensitivity and track how it changed as the study progressed.

The results were remarkable. The tests showed that our participants were physically changing. Based on their laboratory measurements, it was clear that their bodies' cells were becoming more and more sensitive to insulin. By the 14-week point, their insulin sensitivity had improved by 24 percent. In other words, something about the diet reactivated their natural insulin's ability to open cell doors to glucose. What that means, of course, is that the diet was addressing the fundamental problem we see in type 2 diabetes: It was helping glucose get to where it belonged.*

Based on these and other studies, the National Institutes of Health—the research branch of the US government—decided to fund a new study.[8] Working with me on the project were researchers from George Washington University School of Medicine and the University of Toronto and dietitians and physicians working with the Physicians Committee for Responsible Medicine, a nonprofit organization I founded in 1985.

The study included 99 people with type 2 diabetes. For 22 weeks, 49 of them followed a diet that was similar to those we had tested earlier. The diet was vegan—meaning that it included no animal products at all—and was low in fat. Also, while we placed no limits on the amount of carbohydrates our participants could have, we encouraged everyone to be selective about the kinds of carbohydrates they ate. Instead of white bread, we encouraged them to choose rye or pumpernickel. Instead of baking potatoes, we favored sweet potatoes and yams. The remaining 50 participants followed a diet based on the ADA guidelines. Once again, we restricted exercise.

What was happening was that the diet had made their cells more sensitive to insulin's action, so they were able to take in nutrients more quickly. Glucose got out of the blood and into the cells, where more of it could be burned up, so to speak. These calories are released as body heat rather than being stored as body fat. Scientists call this the thermic effect of food, and it provides a small extra edge for weight loss.

Over the ensuing weeks, many participants found their blood sugar falling to the extent that they had to cut back on their diabetes medications. That was a happy outcome, but it was not our goal. In fact, we

---

* The study turned up another particularly remarkable finding. In a laboratory at George Washington University, we measured the participants' metabolism—how fast their bodies burned calories. This was done by measuring how much oxygen they consumed minute by minute and how much carbon dioxide they produced after being given a test meal (two cans of a standard liquid formula).

After 14 weeks on the experimental diet, it was clear that the participants had a significant increase in their after-meal calorie burn; their after-meal calorie-burning speed increased by 16 percent.[9]

were trying to keep medications unchanged as much as we could so we could isolate the effect of the diet on their blood sugar. The combination of the diet and the blood sugar–lowering drugs was so powerful, however, that many participants *had* to reduce their doses or discontinue medications altogether to keep their blood sugar from dropping too low.

To really gauge what the diet could do, we looked at those participants whose medications had stayed constant and how the diet affected A1C—the principal gauge of blood glucose control. The ADA diet had reduced A1C by 0.4 percentage point—a good change. But the vegan diet was three times more effective. It had reduced A1C by 1.2 percentage points (the average person's value fell from 8.0 to 6.8 percent during the 22-week study). That is a stronger effect than is seen with a typical diabetes medication. The vegan diet also proved highly effective in reducing body weight and cholesterol.

To put all this in perspective, the landmark UK Prospective Diabetes Study showed that a 1-point drop in A1C for people with type 2 diabetes lowers the risk of eye or kidney complications by about 37 percent.[10] This is the effect of just the A1C drop without considering the ability of the diet to also reduce cholesterol and blood pressure.[11]

In the next chapter, I will show you how you can test this diet to see what it can do for you. But let's look a bit closer at the science behind this approach.

TOWARD THE PERFECT DIET

Setting aside animal products and keeping oily foods to a minimum may sound challenging, but our participants commonly reported just the opposite. One man, Walter, said, "I'm amazed at how easy it was to adapt to this diet. And I feel great. Within 2 months, I lost 20 pounds. And the more amazing thing to me is that my glucose averages have fallen by 30 to 40 points."

For Mark, the change was "an adventure. I tried new restaurants, new recipes, and different foods I would never have eaten before. My main goal was to lose weight, and I've lost a good 30 pounds so far. When I started, my fasting blood sugar was 260 to 360. And it dropped like a rock. Now I'm between 130 and 135. And I don't get tired in the afternoon like I used to."

Nancy agreed. She felt totally adjusted to the diet within about 30 days. "And within 5 months of making the change," she said, "my blood sugar fell so much that I was able to stop one of my medications. I have much more energy and really feel tremendous."

I will walk you through the diet step by step. If it sounds like a very healthful diet, it certainly is—and not just for controlling blood sugar.

In 1990, Dean Ornish, MD, a young Harvard-trained physician, discovered a remarkable feature of a low-fat, vegetarian diet. He tested the diet in individuals with heart disease and added other healthy life-style changes—regular exercise, stress modification, and smoking cessation. Because the diet contained no animal products, it had no cholesterol at all and very little fat. After a year's time, each patient had a special x-ray of the heart called an angiogram, and Dr. Ornish's team compared the results with angiograms done on the same patients at the beginning of the study. The results made medical history. The patients' coronary arteries, which had been blocked by years of poor diet, were actually starting to open again. The difference was clearly visible in 82 percent of the patients after 1 year. This occurred without surgery or drugs—even without cholesterol-lowering medication.[12, 13]

Other researchers have shown that this same sort of diet change reduces blood pressure. Apparently, eliminating animal fats reduces the viscosity ("thickness") of the blood. That is, the blood becomes less like grease and more like water, so it easily flows through the arteries, causing blood pressure to fall. Blood pressure is also reduced by the potassium in vegetables and fruits, and other characteristics of plant foods augment this benefit.[14]

Vegetarians are slimmer, too. The average person who embraces a vegetarian diet loses about 10 percent of his or her body weight.

These changes would be welcomed by most of us, but if you have diabetes, they can be lifesaving. This is because, as you saw in Chapter 1, persistently high blood sugar can attack the blood vessels of your heart, eyes, kidneys, and legs. What kills most people who have diabetes (that is, those who have not made the diet changes you are reading about) is damage to their hearts. A diet that reverses that process—turning the clock backward on heart disease, reducing blood pressure, and trimming weight—is powerful medicine for everyone with diabetes, whether type 1 or type 2.

Imagine if your eyes were damaged by the disease. An ophthalmologic surgeon, laser in hand, would carefully try to repair your tender retinas. But what if foods could help avert this damage in the first place? A diet change that brings your blood sugar under control, brings your blood pressure down, and helps rejuvenate your arteries gives a measure of respite to the tiny blood vessels in your eyes. It does the same for the tiny vessels that make up the filtering unit in your kidneys, making it less likely that you will ever need dialysis. And of course, it works powerfully inside the heart.

Now, do not misunderstand me. I am not suggesting that you should forgo needed medical treatments and rely on diet alone. But a diet change—if it goes far enough and begins early enough—can revolutionize your health, dramatically cut your risk of complications, and even reverse these complications to a degree.

INSIDE THE CELL

In discussing type 2 diabetes, I have described each cell of the body as being rather like a gummed-up lock. Research has shown this analogy to be surprisingly apt. Indeed, insulin's ability to work is blocked by the accumulation of something within the cells: not gum, but fat.

In the February 12, 2004, issue of the *New England Journal of Medicine,* Yale University researchers reported an amazing discovery.[15] They tested young adults whose parents or grandparents had had type 2 diabetes. All were thin and healthy, and none had diabetes at that point. But some were insulin resistant, meaning that when they were given a test dose of glucose, it built up more than it should have in their bloodstream. The researchers found out why: Inside their muscle cells were tiny amounts of fat, fat that interfered with insulin's

Fat inside Cells Interferes with Insulin's Action

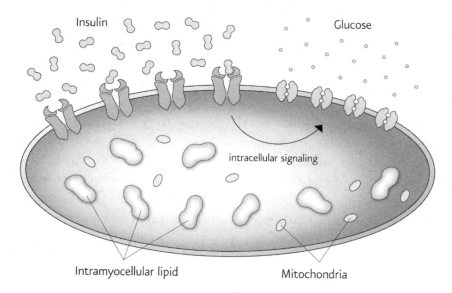

Normally, insulin attaches to receptors on the cell's surface and signals the cell membrane to allow glucose to enter. However, if fat, called intramyocellular lipid, accumulates inside the cell, it interferes with insulin's intracellular signaling process. Tiny organelles, called mitochondria, are supposed to burn fat, and their failure to keep up with the accumulating fat may be the origin of type 2 diabetes. Luckily, evidence shows that diet changes can reduce the amount of fat inside the cell.

ability to work. Their bodies made insulin normally, and it reached their muscle cells with no problem. Once it got there, though, it did not work properly. The muscle cells simply could not fully respond to insulin because they contained bits of fat, like gum jammed in a lock rendering a key useless.

How did this fat get there? Well, muscle cells normally store a tiny amount of fat, which provides an energy source for physical activity. The amount is normally quite small, and the fat simply waits for that day when you are much more active than usual and need a bit of extra energy. For some reason, in these young people, fat had built up much more than it should have—to levels 80 percent higher than in other young people. The fat buildup had reached the point where it was gumming up the lock. That is, it was interfering with the cell's ability to respond to insulin, and that meant that diabetes was very likely in their future unless something changed in a major way.

I should emphasize that the fat inside your cells is different from the fat around your waistline. Even if you are quite slim, you may still be accumulating fat within your muscle cells. The participants in the Yale study *were* slim, averaging only 141 pounds. They were young and healthy. But just as young people who smoke are setting the stage for cancer decades later, young people who accumulate fat inside their muscle cells are paving the way for diabetes.

Until now, diabetes diets have not been designed to alter what goes on inside the cells. Instead, they have been designed to compensate for the problem, so to speak. Because your cells cannot handle glucose— that is, insulin has trouble getting glucose into them—the diets limit sugars and foods that contain carbohydrate, because when carbohydrate is digested, it releases sugars. But what if a change in diet could actually alter the fat buildup within the cells and reverse the trend toward gradually worsening insulin resistance?

I believe this is exactly what we can do—exactly what you *will* do as you make the diet changes described in this book. But first, a few more details from inside the cells.

TINY FURNACES THAT BURN FAT

There is a term for the tiny bits of fat that build up inside muscle cells. Scientists call them intramyocellular lipids (*intra-* means "inside," *myo-* is "muscle," and *lipid* is "fat"—literally, fat inside muscle cells). As you have seen, these traces of fat start accumulating many years before diabetes manifests.[16]

Let's go one step further and look at how the fat builds up. Your cells have microscopic "furnaces" or "burners" that are supposed to metabolize bits of fat and convert it into energy. If all is operating normally, fat enters the cell and these tiny burners use it up. These burners are called mitochondria, and they are responsible for turning fat or other fuel sources into energy to power your muscle cells. If you are steadily accumulating fat, that is a sign that your burners—your mitochondria—are falling down on the job.

In type 2 diabetes, the problem appears to be too few mitochondria. That is, people with type 2 diabetes have fewer mitochondria than they need to burn up the accumulating fat. If they had more of these little "furnaces" inside each cell, things would be very different.

Surprisingly enough, it may be that the number of mitochondria you have depends on what you eat. Let me describe a second research study.

At Pennington Biomedical Research Center in Baton Rouge, Louisiana, researchers studied 10 young men. They averaged just 23 years of age; were reasonably trim, averaging 174 pounds; and were healthy. The researchers put them on a high-fat diet that drew about half its calories from fats.[17] This is much more fat than you would want to have in your diet, but it is not far different from what many people actually eat. After just 3 days on a high-fat diet, the men had accumulated significantly more intramyocellular lipids, so the first lesson of this study was that fat builds up quickly. Depending on the foods you eat, you can pack fat into your cells surprisingly rapidly.

Then the researchers tested the genes that produce mitochondria. Just as you have genes in your cells that allow you to make bones, hormones, skin, hair, and all the other structures of your body, you also have genes that serve as blueprints for mitochondria. It turned out that the fatty foods these volunteers ate did more than just pack fat into their cells; they actually *turned off the genes that would help burn fat.* The genes that produce mitochondria were in fact partially disabled. It was as if the men's bodies were trying to avoid burning the fat they had eaten so they could save it inside the cells for future use.

Imagine what this means: You have eaten fatty foods and, as a result, tiny bits of fat have accumulated in your muscle cells. This fat interferes with the normal workings of the cells, including their ability to respond to insulin. If insulin is unable to work, glucose cannot get into the cells, and it builds up in the bloodstream. Then, those fatty foods actually seem to disable your genes that would produce the mitochondria you need to burn up this accumulating fat. Your ability to eliminate fat inside your cells seems to be slowed down when you eat fatty foods.

Let me speculate about why all this occurs.

Your body chemistry began to take shape many thousands of years ago, long before fast-food restaurants and convenience stores ever got their first shipments of cheese and fryer grease. Our human ancestors did not find fatty foods growing on trees—or at least not many of them. On the rare occasions when they ate fatty foods—meat, eggs, nuts, or avocados, for example—their bodies may actually have tried to save some of the fat from these foods in case they needed it to power their muscles or food became scarce. Thus, it would not be surprising if a sudden influx of fat in the muscle cells signals them to *turn off* the fat-burning mitochondria and save the fat for future needs. Today, of course, that is the last thing we want. We want to power up our mitochondria—turn on those little furnaces to eliminate fat.

Well, can you get rid of this fat? Let's say you stopped eating fatty foods. Would intramyocellular lipid start to disappear?

Let me share the results of a startling experiment. At Catholic University in Rome, Italy, eight patients underwent gastric bypass surgery.[18] The operation is commonly done as a last-ditch treatment for massive obesity, and for good reason. What it involves is this: The stomach is stapled so that only a tiny pouch about the size of an egg is left to receive food. Then the intestine is cut in two. The first part of the intestine simply lies unused, while the lower portion of the small intestine is attached directly to the tiny stomach pouch. In this way, the patient cannot eat much food, and there is much less intestine available to absorb the nutrients from whatever food is eaten.

After the procedure, the patients were essentially starving. They could eat very little food at any given meal, and any fats they ate were poorly absorbed because the first part of the small intestine, which is where fats are absorbed, was no longer connected to the stomach.

As you might imagine, they lost weight, dropping from an average of more than 300 pounds (137 kg) to 229 pounds (104 kg) in the first 6 months. That is not unusual after such drastic surgery. What was striking was the effect on their cells. The fat inside their muscle cells—their intramyocellular lipid—dropped by 87 percent. And even though they were still overweight, their insulin resistance had largely disappeared.

I am not recommending that you have this procedure. I am presenting these findings to make a critically important point: The fat inside your cells is not a permanent fixture. If the influx of fat stops, the fat inside the cells dissipates, and when that happens, *the cells start to regain their normal function.*

Surgery is a drastic solution, but the Italian researchers also tested whether a low-calorie diet without surgery could deplete intramyocellular lipid—and it did. Following a 1,200-calorie diet for 6 months, the patients lost about 30 pounds on average and eliminated about 8 percent of the fat inside their cells. Now, that modest result came from a diet that focused just on cutting calories rather than on eating particular *types* of food, which will be the focus of this program. The next step is to make the diet more powerful so it works a little more like surgery, without all the obvious risks of an operation.

Let's go a step further. At Imperial College School of Medicine in London, researchers studied a group of individuals following a vegan diet. They compared the participants to others who were similar in age and body weight but were not following a vegan diet.[19] When the researchers measured the intramyocellular lipid in each participant's calf muscles, they found it was 31 percent lower in the vegans than in the omnivores. It looks as if there is something about the diet that helps prevent fat buildup in cells.

These studies show—loudly and clearly—that the accumulation of fat in the cells and all the problems it causes are not simply a matter of genes. Genes do play a role, but these effects are very much a matter of diet, too, and *it can change dramatically.*

In Part 2, you will see how to select foods to address this problem in the most powerful way possible.

CHAPTER 3

A Revolution in Type 1 Diabetes

If you have type 1 diabetes, the diet changes you will soon learn about can be lifesaving. No doubt you have heard that type 1 diabetes increases the risk of heart problems and other complications. When you really take control, however, all these risks plummet.

Research has proven that you are not powerless against the complications of diabetes. There is a lot you can do to protect yourself.

The Diabetes Control and Complications Trial did it with medication. The study was sponsored by the US government and included 1,441 people with type 1 diabetes. Some of the participants took insulin once or twice daily, as is common practice. The remaining participants were asked to follow a more intensive program. They took insulin three or four times daily, either by injection or via an insulin pump. They checked their blood glucose several times a day and adjusted their insulin doses accordingly. Over 17 years of follow-up, the extra care these individuals took paid off dramatically. Careful tracking of blood sugar and medication adjustments lowered the risk of heart problems by 50 percent.[1]

Also, although people with diabetes are at risk for eye problems, careful blood glucose control reduced that risk by 76 percent compared to people on traditional medical therapy. It cut the risk of kidney problems by 39 percent and reduced the risk of neuropathy by 60 percent.[2]

The study treatment involved medication rather than diet, but it proved a vitally important point. Many people had imagined that diabetes complications are simply inevitable; this study showed otherwise. Gaining control over your blood glucose makes an enormous difference. Now, with type 1 diabetes, you will need to use insulin to achieve that goal. But diet and exercise offer additional power that too few people take advantage of. And diet is the focus of this book.

Also, it is important to understand that blood sugar control—as vital as it is—is just one part of the equation. Your risk of developing problems with your heart, kidneys, eyes, or extremities also depends on your blood pressure, cholesterol levels, and other factors. The goal now is to adjust your diet to control all of these to the extent that we can, adding medications as necessary according to your doctor's advice.

TOWARD AN OPTIMAL LIFESTYLE

In type 1 diabetes, your greatest risk is to your heart and blood vessels. If you do nothing, cardiovascular disease lies in wait. In fact, it strikes the majority of people with type 1 diabetes. We now have a better understanding than ever before about how to use diet and lifestyle changes to protect the heart, not only for people with diabetes but for anyone. Chapters 4 and 5 will cover how and what to eat in great detail, and Chapters 12 and 13 will discuss the complications head-on. In the meantime, here are the keys.

A healthy diet. Follow the diet steps outlined in the next chapter. These practices eliminate cholesterol and animal fat, keep fats in general very low, and guide you away from sugar and refined carbohydrates and toward healthy complex carbohydrates.

As you will see, there is a special advantage to a vegetarian diet, or I should say a *vegan* diet—meaning a menu that includes no animal products at all. Dietary cholesterol is found only in animal products.*

---

*It is a good idea to eliminate cholesterol from your diet completely. There is no "good" cholesterol in foods. Rather, cholesterol in foods always tends to increase your blood cholesterol level. This is in contrast to cholesterol that is measured by blood tests, which doctors separate into "good" (HDL) cholesterol and "bad" (LDL) cholesterol, among other forms. HDL cholesterol is "good" because it is leaving the body.

Animal products also tend to be high in the saturated ("bad") fats that tend to cause your body to make additional cholesterol, an effect that is actually much greater than eating cholesterol itself. A plant-based diet eliminates these problems. It has another major benefit as well: It derives its protein from plants rather than from animal products. Research studies have shown that among people with any degree of kidney damage, animal protein increases the risk of further kidney deterioration.[3] On the other hand, healthy beans, grains, and vegetables are just what your kidneys ordered.

A plant-based diet does more than reduce your risk of complications. It may also reduce the amount of insulin you need. When people with type 1 diabetes begin a low-fat, vegan diet, many report that their insulin requirements fall dramatically. Although the reasons for this are not entirely clear, it is a very welcome result.

Please read the next chapters very carefully. They will show you how to begin.

No smoking. If you smoke, now is the time to stop. If you have tried 50 times, it is time for try number 51. You can and will succeed. Ask your doctor to help you.

Regular exercise. Even modest exercise, such as daily walking, makes a big difference. See your doctor, who will assess your heart, your joints, and your overall health to make sure you are ready for exercise. See Chapter 11 for ways to get started.

Stress management. Stress affects your health directly, causing fight-or-flight hormones to flood into your bloodstream. In turn, these hormones typically raise your blood sugar. Stress also disrupts your eating routines and interferes with sleep.

Getting a handle on stress does not mean stepping back from the challenges of life. It means finding ways to enjoy life fully without letting stress get out of control. There are many healthy ways to relax, including meditation, yoga, and even simple breathing exercises.

As you saw in the previous chapter, Dr. Dean Ornish showed that these four steps—a healthy vegetarian diet, smoking cessation, regular exercise, and stress management—can actually reverse heart disease, even without the use of cholesterol-lowering medications. That is a tremendous benefit. Your doctor may add medications to your regimen to protect you further.

These lifestyle changes will not eliminate the need to use insulin for type 1 diabetes. But they can help you stay healthy, minimizing the effects of diabetes on your life.

A NEW UNDERSTANDING OF THE CAUSES OF TYPE 1 DIABETES

Let's think for a moment beyond improving the health of people with type 1 diabetes. What if we could actually prevent it in the first place? Research over the past 3 decades suggests that we may already have the ability to prevent many cases of type 1 diabetes.

If you thought the disease was simply genetic and there was no way to stop it, read on. Studies of identical twins have set that notion aside. Identical twins, of course, have exactly the same genes, so they have the same hair color, eye color, and facial features. If a disease were simply genetic, then both twins would have it. But type 1 diabetes does not work that way. As I mentioned in Chapter 1, if one twin has diabetes, the other has less than a 40 percent chance of developing it.

So, although genes play a role, it is clear that type 1 diabetes is not simply a genetic disease. Something else triggers it—something in the child's early environment.

For many years, researchers have known that type 1 diabetes occurs when the immune system attacks and destroys the insulin-producing cells in the pancreas. Your immune system, of course, is your defense against viruses, bacteria, and cancer cells. It is not supposed to attack your own healthy body tissues, but that is exactly what occurs in type 1 diabetes.

To understand why this happens, let's look at a few basics. The complex defense network of your immune system is made up of specialized white blood cells. Some of these cells engulf invading germs and digest them. Others make antibodies—molecules that attach to invading organisms like harpoons and identify them for other immune cells to attack. If you have type 1 diabetes, your immune system has made a major error: It has attacked and destroyed your insulin-producing cells, resulting in what scientists call an autoimmune disease.

But why does it occur? Back in 1992, a team of Canadian and Finnish researchers reported an important discovery in the *New England Journal of Medicine*. Examining blood samples from 142 children newly diagnosed with type 1 diabetes, they found that each of the children had antibodies that were primed to attack cow's milk proteins. These antibodies had apparently arisen in response to cow proteins in their infant formula, but the antibodies were also capable of attacking the body's insulin-producing cells.[4] It turned out that a portion of the cow's milk protein was biochemically an exact match for a portion of human insulin-producing cells. The antibodies that arose to destroy the cow's milk protein ended up attacking the children's insulin-producing cells. The pancreatic cells were destroyed by "friendly fire."

This study and others suggested a scenario that could lead to type 1 diabetes. It has long been known that when a very young infant is fed cow's milk formula, some of the milk proteins pass from the digestive tract into the bloodstream.[5, 6] It is possible that the infant's immune system recognizes these bovine proteins as foreign and forms antibodies to attack them and that these antibodies attack not only the cow proteins but also the insulin-producing cells of the pancreas. This destructive process is presumably gradual; when nearly all the insulin-producing cells are gone, type 1 diabetes results. The researchers believed that the mature digestive tracts of adults would not allow these dairy proteins to pass through the intestinal wall and into the bloodstream, but in infants, the molecules passed through more easily.

The study suggested that one way to prevent type 1 diabetes, at least for many children, might be to avoid exposure to cow's milk early in life. Needless to say, in the early 1990s, neither parents nor pediatricians had any idea about this. Cow's milk formulas were routinely fed to infants, and they still are. When children are not breastfed, some sort of formula has to be used. And while some children are given soy formulas that would presumably pose no diabetes risk, many are given cow's milk varieties.

In 1992, when the *New England Journal of Medicine* report emerged, the well-known baby doctor Benjamin Spock, MD, and I held a press conference. We were joined by Frank Oski, MD, director of pediatrics at Johns Hopkins University, and other nutrition experts. We recommended that parents be given information about the potential risks of early exposure to cow's milk. After all, parents are pushed very hard to give cow's milk to their children, but they rarely hear of potential risks it might pose. We called for an end to recommendations that push milk consumption on children and said that parents should have good information in order to decide what to feed their children.

The event proved controversial. Most major newspapers and broadcast channels covered the story. The American Medical Association (AMA) sharply criticized Dr. Spock and me for casting doubt on the healthfulness of dairy products. Research teams trying to replicate these findings got mixed results, with some coming up empty-handed. Still other researchers pointed out that finding the antibodies required special techniques, without which the antibodies would remain elusive.[7] Eventually, the American Academy of Pediatrics convened a work group to look into the matter. Two years later, in 1994, the group issued a report. Based on more than 90 studies, the group agreed that indeed, the risk of diabetes can very likely be reduced if infants are not exposed to cow's milk proteins early in life.[8] Eventually, the AMA withdrew its objections.

While Dr. Spock and I felt there was already substantial evidence and good reason to issue cautions about exposure to dairy products early in life, the controversy did not end there. There was only one way to know whether dairy proteins could actually incite the series of events leading to type 1 diabetes: The theory had to be put to the test. A European team began that process.

TESTING THE DAIRY-DIABETES THEORY

In a pilot study, researchers in Finland, Sweden, and Estonia identified 242 newborns at risk for developing type 1 diabetes—each had a first-degree relative with the condition. The researchers then encouraged their mothers to breastfeed. When mothers were ready to wean their infants, the researchers asked half to use a specially modified baby formula in which dairy proteins were broken up into individual amino acids—protein building blocks that are too small to elicit an immune reaction. The other families were allowed to use a regular cow's milk formula. The research aimed to see whether avoiding exposure to intact cow's milk proteins could reduce the likelihood of developing diabetes.[9]

As the years went by, the researchers found that the children who were fed the special formula were much less likely to develop the dangerous antibodies. In fact, the risk of developing antibodies to their insulin-producing cells was cut by 62 percent.

The study was small, only a pilot trial, but it did follow most of the children through their first 6 to 8 years of life. During those years, several children developed diabetes. Of those receiving unmodified formula, eight developed the disease, and in the modified-formula group, five developed it. As it turned out, two of those five had dropped out of the study right at the start and never actually received the modified formula. That meant that only three children in the modified-formula group developed diabetes, compared to eight in the regular-formula group. The study suggested that the cow's milk theory may well be part of the puzzle, but it was too small to be definitive, and the research team began a much larger test in 2002 involving families in 15 countries.

There were some limitations to this pilot study. First, it restricted dairy consumption only during the first several months of life. It is not clear whether later exposure, say, at 8 or 9 months of age, might put some children at risk as well. After all, it has long been known that very large dairy protein molecules can sometimes pass from the digestive tract into the bloodstream, even in adults. The study did not address whether exposure to dairy proteins could trigger type 1 diabetes in children who are beyond early infancy.

Second, the study did not ask breastfeeding mothers to avoid cow's milk in their own diets. For decades, we have known that some cow's milk proteins ingested by a nursing mother end up in her breast milk. They come from her digestive tract, are absorbed into her bloodstream, and find their way into the breast milk, sometimes making babies colicky.[10] Thus, in order to avoid exposing babies to dairy proteins, it is important to eliminate them not only from infants' diets but also from the diets of their breastfeeding mothers.

One last caution about this study: It did not actually exclude dairy products from the children's diets. Rather, it used a milk product treated to break up the dairy proteins. If anything in milk other than these proteins contributes to the problem, this study would not have been able to detect it. Even so, it was an important step in coming to understand how parts of an infant's diet may lead to diabetes.

The study illuminated other contributors to diabetes, too. Prior evidence had suggested that viral infections may play a role, and indeed, viruses appear to have done so for some infants in the milk study. Specifically, viruses seem to stimulate immune cells, perhaps making them more active against cow's milk proteins than they would normally be. Or, cow's milk proteins may influence the course of viral infections in some way.[11] The idea is that the interplay between cow's milk formula and viruses may put babies at increased risk.

No one knows what the research on milk and type 1 diabetes will ultimately show. If the theory turns out to be correct, it suggests that avoiding cow's milk products, at least during the first several months of life, could greatly reduce the likelihood of developing this disease.

Needless to say, breastfeeding instead of feeding formula poses no risks for children. Quite the opposite: Breastfed babies gain many advantages, including better overall health and even a few extra IQ points, compared to their formula-fed counterparts. And the most healthful breastfeeding is done when mothers follow a diet free of foods that can harm their babies.

Other risk factors for diabetes may yet emerge in research studies. And for children who are already in the midst of an antibody attack, researchers are studying means of intervening to try to stop the destruction of their insulin-producing cells.

STAYING HEALTHY

If we are able to prevent diabetes, we will have a very powerful tool at our disposal. For people who already have type 1 diabetes, there are effective steps they can take to help them stay healthy. Keeping blood glucose under control is essential, and stabilizing cholesterol levels and blood pressure protects the heart and blood vessels. The same sort of diet that is described in this book for type 2 diabetes is likely to be enormously beneficial for people with type 1 as well, helping them to prevent complications and reduce their insulin doses.

PART 2

The Program

CHAPTER 4

A Powerful
New Menu

We are setting our sights on a dramatically better result than previous diets could deliver—a result that's possible through a new approach to eating that I will explain in this chapter. If you have type 2 diabetes, you do not want to cater to insulin resistance; you want to counteract it. If you have type 1 diabetes, you want to get your blood sugar under good control, minimize your medications, and stay in good health. This chapter will show you the principles of revolutionizing your menu. Then, in the following chapters, I will show you how to put them to work as you plan your meals.

For type 2 diabetes, our goal is to "clean the gum out of the locks." As you recall, the fundamental problem in type 2 diabetes appears to be the accumulation of tiny amounts of fat inside muscle cells. They make it hard for insulin to do its job by blocking what is called insulin signaling. That is, they interfere with the process by which insulin opens the cell membrane to allow glucose to enter. You need to select foods that reverse this process.

A diet revamp can also help protect your body from the disease process. That is crucial for both type 1 and type 2 diabetes.

As you will see, these diet changes are far-reaching and powerful. You may also find, as many of our study participants did, that learning the plan's guidelines is a simple process. There are no limits on portions, calories, or carbohydrates. You will focus on *what you eat*, so *how much you eat* generally takes care of itself. But we are getting ahead of ourselves.

Let's first look at the menu changes that make the diet so effective. Then, in the following chapter, I will walk you through various ways to adopt them to make this diet doable for you.

To reverse the course of diabetes, "clean the gum out of the locks," and allow the heart and blood vessels the best chance of reversing any existing blockages, there are three guidelines.

1. Set aside animal products.
2. Keep vegetable oils to a minimum.
3. Favor foods with a low Glycemic Index.

Now, there is no need to panic. I know this sounds like a tall order. I am going to walk you through each step to show you the whys and hows. Soon, it will be second nature. For now, I just want you to understand the principles.

1. SET ASIDE ANIMAL PRODUCTS

There are two possible sources of fat in the diet: animal products and vegetable oils. This guideline tackles the first of these.

Needless to say, if you are not eating beef, you will not get any beef fat. If you are not eating chicken, you will not get any chicken fat. Following this guideline means purging the animal fat from your diet. The program you are about to start omits meat, dairy products, and eggs.

As you saw in Chapter 2, researchers who measured the fat inside the muscle cells of people on high-fat diets showed that the fat you eat can rapidly increase the amount of fat in your cells. Exactly the opposite appears to happen in people who avoid animal products. As you recall, people following a vegan diet had 31 percent less intracellular fat compared with people on a regular diet.[1] That means improved insulin sensitivity. That is a great start, and the next guidelines are designed to carry you further.

You will get another benefit. When you set aside animal products, you do more than free yourself from animal fat; since animal products are the only source of cholesterol in the diet, leaving them off your plate also eliminates all the cholesterol from your diet. As your cells reclaim their health, the rest of your body does, too.

Instead of eggs and bacon for breakfast, you might have a big bowl of old-fashioned oatmeal with cinnamon or blueberries, half a cantaloupe, and some rye toast. Perhaps you might add some veggie sausage or veggie bacon.

For lunch, instead of, say, meat chili, you might have veggie chili or hearty lentil soup. If you generally go for a burger, you might choose a veggie burger. If you have dinner at an Italian restaurant, you might have spaghetti with tomato sauce, wild mushrooms, artichoke hearts, and fresh basil. At a Mexican restaurant, you would skip the meat taco in favor of a bean burrito (hold the cheese) or veggie

Ready for a Change

In one of our research studies, half the volunteers were assigned to a low-fat vegan diet, and the other half were instructed to follow a more conventional diet for diabetes. Since it was to be an unbiased test, the diet assignment was done by a computer. So the process was random, and neither the volunteers nor we had any influence over who got which diet. Nonetheless, I was curious about how the volunteers felt about the two diets, so I asked them. If there had been an opportunity to choose one of the diets, which one would they have chosen? I expected most to say they would have chosen the conventional diet—it is familiar to most people who have been diagnosed with diabetes, and I thought the volunteers might feel a bit of trepidation about giving up meat and dairy products.

As it turned out, their preferences were just the opposite. *The volunteers actually preferred the vegan diet by about two to one.* The reason, I learned, was that many had already been on a conventional diet and had found it dull and not very effective. Many of them had heard about the advantages of a vegan diet. Others had relatives who followed a vegetarian or vegan diet, and they wanted to give it a try.

Both groups embraced their assignments. Some did well on the conventional diet and some did not. The results with the vegan diet, however, were powerful and consistent.

fajitas. At a Chinese restaurant, you could have your pick of the many vegetable dishes on a bed of rice.

At this point, you may be thinking, "Spaghetti? Rice? Am I allowed to have these carbohydrate-rich foods?" The answer is yes. Now, I know that people with diabetes have heard over and over that they must limit rice, pasta, and other starchy foods. But keep in mind that diabetes—and overweight—has been rare in countries that have made these foods their staples. The plan does have guidelines about carbohydrates, but they relate mainly to which ones are the best choices, not how much you put on your plate. In our studies, we have found that people who include plenty of healthy carbohydrates in their diets do *better*, not worse.

"I can understand omitting beef," you may say, "but why eliminate chicken and fish?" Well, the nutritional makeup of these foods may surprise you. They have significant amounts of fat and cholesterol, and they lack the fiber and healthy carbohydrate you need.

Chicken, of course, is where chicken fat comes from. Even if you strip away the skin and eat only white meat, about 23 percent of the calories come from fat. Much of that fat is the "bad" form—*saturated* fat, the kind that pushes your cholesterol upward and worsens insulin resistance.

What a Difference: Animal versus Plant Foods					
	FAT (% OF CALORIES)	CHOLESTEROL (MG)		FAT (% OF CALORIES)	CHOLESTEROL (MG)
Salmon, Atlantic	40	71	Apple	3	0
Beef, bottom round, lean*	33	86	Beans, navy	4	0
Chicken, white meat, skinless	23	85	Broccoli	11	0
Pork loin, lean	41	81	Lentils	3	0
Trout, rainbow	35	69	Orange	4	0
Tuna, white	21	42	Rice, brown	7	0

*Meat servings are 3.5 ounces (100 grams).

SOURCE: USDA, Agricultural Research Service Nutrient Data Laboratory, https://ndb.nal.usda.gov/ndb/search/list, accessed April 8, 2017.

Fish vary. Some types are lower in fat than chicken, while others, such as salmon, are quite high. But all fish have fat, and much of it—between 15 and 30 percent—is saturated fat. All fish have cholesterol, too. Some, such as shrimp and lobster, are much higher in cholesterol, ounce for ounce, than steak.

Of course, some people eat fish precisely *because* it has fat in it. That is, a portion of the fat in fish is in the omega-3 form. Omega-3 fats are reputed to block the formation of blood clots that could lead to heart attacks.

Scientific evidence has not been supportive. In large, carefully conducted research studies, fish oils have not been shown to protect the heart. They do not reduce the likelihood of a heart attack or stroke or reduce the risk of dying. They do not help healthy people who are trying to avert their first heart attack, and they do not work for people who have already had a heart attack and are trying to avoid another one.[2, 3]

Could the supposed benefits of omega-3s be just a fish story? Well, it is important to remember that fish fats are mixtures, just as all fats are. Fish oils do indeed contain some omega-3 fat, but they also contain plenty of saturated fat. As noted above, from 15 to 30 percent of the fat in fish is plain old saturated fat. That's less than in beef (about 50 percent) or chicken (about 30 percent), but it is considerably more than you need. There is no specific need for saturated fat in your diet at all.

The load of fat in fish might explain the disconcerting fact that fish consumption is linked to a higher risk of developing diabetes. In 2009, the American Diabetes Association reported in its journal, *Diabetes Care,* that people who regularly ate fish, but no other meats, had a 4.8 percent prevalence of diabetes, compared to 3.2 percent for lacto-ovo-vegetarians and 2.9 percent for vegans.[4] In other words, having fish in your diet does not help; it actually increases diabetes risk.

Similarly, Harvard researchers found that people who ate the most fish had a 24 percent higher risk of developing diabetes, compared with those who generally avoided fish.[5]

Finally, if you are looking to lose weight, it is important to note that "good fats" pack in just as many calories as "bad fats." That is to say, omega-3s are every bit as fattening as any other fat or oil. All fats and oils have 9 calories in every gram, compared with only 4 calories per gram of carbohydrate.

In practice, chicken-and-fish diets are routinely disappointing. We have carefully tested these diets and found that, even when they are followed very closely, their ability to reduce LDL ("bad") cholesterol is only about half that of a plant-based (vegan) diet, and their ability to control blood sugar or blood pressure or to help you lose weight is limited, too.[6]

Much more effective are diets that eliminate animal products altogether. Our studies and those of other researchers have shown that plant-based diets cut LDL cholesterol far more effectively than any other diet approach.

Now, you will notice that when you avoid animal products, your diet is not just free of animal fat; it is also free of animal *protein*. That is important because animal protein can harm the kidneys, and protecting them is a key goal. Protein from plant sources is the way to go.

If life without chicken or cheese sounds challenging, take heart from the experiences of the folks who participated in our research. They found the transition to be smooth. They found tastes they liked better than their old go-to foods. And within a few weeks, they were very much in charge—not only of their menus but also of their health. They found that excess weight was already starting to melt away, their blood sugar was coming under control, their cholesterol levels were falling, and very soon, many started to cut back on—or even discontinue—their medications.

How Nancy and Vance Did It

How did Nancy and Vance, whom you met in the Introduction, fare with the diet changes?

For Nancy, the change was a welcome one. She was fed up with the lack of results from the previous diet she had been given and thought a vegan diet sounded like a good approach. She wanted to lose weight, and she was sick of feeling so low on energy. This, she hoped, might be an answer.

Nancy grew up in Minnesota. Her mother was not an especially talented cook, she says, but her Scandinavian family loved food. Her mother and sisters all struggled with weight problems.

Like most of our study volunteers, Nancy had already made healthy changes to her diet over the years. She had stopped eating beef, ate plenty of vegetables, and had gotten away from fatty dressings, so making the shift was reasonably easy.

As she began the study, she started her day with oatmeal topped with cinnamon and fat-free vanilla soy milk. At midmorning, she liked to have a snack, usually fruit such as apples, bananas, raspberries, blueberries, grapes, or oranges.

For lunch, she had a hearty vegan soup such as minestrone, vegetable soup, sweet potato soup, or chili, along with a salad made with fresh spinach; tomatoes; red, yellow, and orange bell peppers; kidney beans and chickpeas; and other ingredients. Her afternoon snack was often fruit, rye crackers, baked tortilla chips with salsa, or hummus and pita bread.

After a long day at work, Nancy had no interest in preparing a gourmet meal, so her dinners were quick and easy: a veggie burger with frozen mixed vegetables, which she microwaved. Sometimes she had nothing more than a bowl of bran cereal. A late-night fruit snack rounded things out.

We gave her group a supermarket tour and provided cooking demonstrations to introduce everyone to healthful products that might be new to them. Nancy preferred to keep it simple and started making a large pot of soup to eat all week. "I am not a cook," she said. "And I find it very easy to stay on this program."

Vance usually started his day with oatmeal, either plain or with apples and cinnamon. He also had toast and fresh fruit. Lunch or dinner was pasta or burritos along with fresh vegetables and fruits. Sometimes his taste called for salads, usually dressed up with beans, blood oranges, or other additions.

"I had to learn to read labels," he said. "It is easy to underestimate the amount of fat or sugar in a can of food. A label might show 6 grams of fat, and you might think that means the whole can. But it actually means just one serving."

For Vance, the vegan diet was the way to go. "I don't have the personality that would let me have just a small piece of chicken or a small piece of beef," he explained. "I have to cut it out altogether. For me, this is a lifestyle change."

THE POWER PLATE

For starters, let me introduce you to the Power Plate, a simple meal-planning guide that my colleagues and I developed. The idea is simple: Build your diet from four healthy staples—whole grains, legumes, vegetables, and fruits.

On your plate, these simple ingredients might translate into a hearty sweet potato chowder, spinach lasagna, Cuban black beans and Spanish rice, lentil and carrot soup, and endless other possibilities. But let's first take a look at the staple foods themselves. These are the ingredients that build healthful meals.

The whole grain group. This group includes brown rice, oats, barley, corn, and all the products that are made from whole grains: breads, cereals, pasta, and many others. In countries where grains are staples, diabetes is much less common than it is in North America and Europe. This should be no surprise: Whole grains are filling but have very little fat and no cholesterol. When selecting grains, let the Glycemic Index guide you to the best choices.

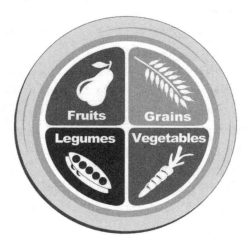

The legume group. This category includes beans, peas, and lentils. It also includes the endless array of soy products, from veggie burgers to meatless hot dogs, tofu, tempeh, miso, and every conceivable kind of deli slice. Legumes are hearty, high-protein foods with a remarkably low GI. They are rich in calcium, iron, and cholesterol-lowering soluble fiber. Whether you favor a chickpea salad, black bean chili, or a soy-based veggie burger or other meat substitute, legumes are handy and healthy.

The one thing the bean group lacks is good public relations. Its health benefits have gone largely unnoticed. Nutrition scientists, however, know that putting these healthy powerhouses front and center on your menu is a great way to drive down your weight, blood sugar, and cholesterol. The US government's National Nutrition and Health Examination Survey showed that people who included beans in their regular menu weighed, on average, 6.5 pounds less than people who generally neglected this healthy food group.[7] The trend showed up in teenagers, too. Teenage bean lovers weighed 7 pounds less and had waistlines that were nearly an inch slimmer compared with their bean-avoiding peers.[8]

Researchers at the University of Toronto confirmed that people who include a serving of beans, chickpeas, lentils, or peas in their daily routine are indeed thinner and have lower levels of LDL ("bad") cholesterol.[9, 10]

If you are new to bean dishes, go easy at first, keep portions modest, and cook them thoroughly. They are likely to cause some gassiness until your digestive tract adapts.

The vegetable group. Each member of the vegetable group is robustly healthful. The green vegetables—asparagus, broccoli, spinach, kale, Swiss chard, and many others—are packed with iron and, except for spinach, high in absorbable calcium. Orange vegetables—carrots, yams, and butternut squash, among others—are loaded with beta-carotene, a cancer fighter. Be generous with them.

Instead of the neglected little pile of overcooked vegetables some people park on their plates, have two or even three different vegetables with your dinner. One of my favorite combinations is "orange plus green," as in mashed butternut squash and broccoli. Sometimes I cook them up fresh, and other times, I simply use frozen. The colors contrast, as does the sweetness of the squash with the heartier flavor of

Grapefruit Interacts with Medications

Surprising as it sounds, if you are on certain medications, you may need to avoid grapefruit.[11] A serving of grapefruit or a glass of grapefruit juice can measurably increase the blood concentrations of drugs you may be taking, to the point of toxicity. Here's how it works: Let's say you were to swallow a cholesterol-lowering drug, like atorvastatin (Lipitor). Normally, enzymes in your intestinal tract and liver will inactivate some of it, reducing the amount that is actively circulating in your blood. This is entirely normal, and your dose was determined with that in mind.

But grapefruit knocks out these drug-limiting enzymes. As a result, you end up with more of the active drug in your bloodstream. About half of all oral medications are metabolized by these enzymes, and even one serving of grapefruit has an effect that lasts all day.

For cholesterol-lowering drugs, this is an issue for atorvastatin (Lipitor), simvastatin (Zocor), and lovastatin (Mevacor), but not for pravastatin (Pravachol), rosuvastatin (Crestor), or fluvastatin (Lescol), because they are metabolized differently.

Grapefruit does the same for dozens of other drugs. So if you have a taste for grapefruit, check with your doctor about how it might interact with any medications you are taking. The same effect comes from limes, Seville oranges (used to make marmalade), and pomelos, but not from typical navel or Valencia oranges. The problem occurs only with oral medications, not injectables.

broccoli. You do not have to be a gourmet chef. Even the most hurried person has time to open a package of frozen vegetables and steam or microwave them.

These foods are loaded with vitamins and minerals, are very low in fat, and like all plant foods, have no cholesterol at all.

Virtually all have healthy low GIs. The main exception is baking potatoes, so favor sweet potatoes instead.

The fruit group. Fruits are loaded with vitamins and, of course, have essentially no fat or cholesterol. Many people with diabetes imagine that because fruits are sweet, they will raise blood sugar. The fact is, though, that nearly all fruits—apples, bananas, blueberries, cherries, clementines, oranges, peaches, pears, and most others—have low GIs.

For a simple and beautiful dessert, combine blueberries with chopped mango, papaya, or banana. You'll think of many other great combinations.

How many servings should you have from each group? You can vary your serving sizes as much as you like. If you prefer Mediterranean cuisine, your plate may be rich in vegetables and pasta. If Asian food is your thing, your plate may hold generous portions of rice or other grains. If you love Latin American foods, you might go for bean dishes. If you come from a typical North American background, you will probably want a variety of all four. In the next chapter, I will show you some easy, delicious ways to get started.

It goes without saying that the recommended foods do not include meat, dairy products, eggs, or greasy fried foods.

Other Permitted Foods

- Fat-free salad dressings and other fat-free condiments

- Coffee (with fat-free nondairy creamer, if desired)

- Occasionally, alcoholic beverages

- Rarely, sugar, nuts, seeds, dark chocolate (made without milk), full-fat soy products such as tofu, tempeh, soy cheese, etc.

Foods to Avoid

- Meats, poultry, fish, eggs (whites and yolks), and all dairy products (regular and fat-free), including milk, yogurt, cheese, ice cream, cream, sour cream, butter, etc.

- Added oils, such as margarine, salad dressings, mayonnaise, cooking oils, etc.

- Fried foods, such as potato chips, french fries, onion rings, doughnuts, etc.

- Avocados, olives, and peanut butter

- Foods with high GIs, such as white bread or white potatoes

Vitamin B_{12} and Vitamin D

Although foods will give you most of the nutrition you need, two supplements are important: vitamin B_{12} and vitamin D. Vitamin B_{12} is essential for healthy nerves and healthy blood, and vitamin D is important for

Soup Nirvana

Walter arrived at one of our research meetings to announce that he had found the perfect lunch. His local supermarket stocks a line of soups from the Tabatchnick company that happen to come in several low-fat vegan varieties, such as black bean soup, split pea soup, and vegetarian chili. With simple, natural ingredients, a serving has about 200 calories and just a gram or two of fat. They are available in both regular and low-sodium versions. Since they are frozen, they keep more or less indefinitely and can be microwaved to make a meal in minutes.

There are also many other great brands, including Dr. McDougall's, Health Valley, and Amy's, that are easy, quick, and healthful.

your bones and may reduce cancer risk. All typical multivitamins contain both and are very convenient. But because multivitamins also have ingredients you may not want (e.g., iron and copper), you can instead just pick up these two vitamins at any drugstore or health food store. You'll find more details in Chapter 10.

Healthier Substitutes for Dairy Products

It may surprise you to learn that some of the biggest sources of fat are lurking in the dairy section. Milk, cheese, and ice cream once enjoyed a healthful reputation that few people questioned, but that has changed. It has become clear that these foods are actually the largest source of saturated ("bad") fat in the diet, and also contribute cholesterol, animal protein, and, in the case of fat-free varieties, a big load of lactose sugar.

Here's the lowdown on dairy, followed by the good news about how easy it is to replace it.

Dairy fat. Cow's milk derives, believe it or not, 49 percent of its calories from fat. That is a lot by any standard. You may imagine that 2 percent milk is much lower in fat. Not so. That 2 percent figure refers to fat content *by weight*, which is deceptive because it is thrown off by milk's water content. When you drink a glass of milk, your body absorbs that water. What matters for your health is how much fat you are left with. Nutritionists look for the *percentage of calories* that come from fat because that figure is unaffected by water content. It turns out that for 2 percent milk, about 35 percent of calories come from nothing but fat.

What is particularly worrisome about milk, though, is the *type* of fat it contains. Most of it is saturated fat, the very kind that is linked to insulin resistance and raises cholesterol levels. Dairy products are actually the leading source of saturated fat in the diet.

Typical yogurt, ice cream, and sour cream products are high in fat, too. Cheese is loaded with it. Many brands derive about 70 percent of their calories from fat.

Dairy sugar. Fat-free dairy products have had their fat removed, but what's still there may surprise you. When the fat is skimmed away, the predominant nutrient in milk is actually sugar—lactose, the dairy sugar.

The lactose molecule is a combination of two smaller sugars, glucose and galactose. Approximately 55 percent of the calories in fat-free milk come from lactose. People who quite rightly avoid sodas and other sugary drinks because of their sugar content will want to be aware that milk products are a major source of sugar, too.

Lactose, of course, is the sugar that causes digestive upset for many people. Lactose intolerance is a normal condition that occurs when the enzymes that allow babies to digest mother's milk naturally start to dissipate. When these enzymes are gone, lactose passes through the intestinal tract undigested. In the lower intestinal tract, bacteria start to ferment the sugar, causing gas, cramps, and diarrhea. Lactose intolerance was once thought to be an abnormality but is now known to be the biological norm. The symptoms come on gradually, sometime after early childhood, and they are simply a sign that you have successfully passed the age of weaning.

Dairy proteins. These proteins have come under scrutiny for their potential contribution to type 1 diabetes, as described in Chapter 3, but they are implicated in many other health concerns as well. Animal proteins appear to accelerate the gradual loss of kidney function that can occur in diabetes.[12] Plant sources of protein—beans, grains, vegetables, and soy products, for example—do not appear to cause this problem.

People who have migraines often report improvement when they avoid certain foods, and milk and other dairy products are often at the top of the list. The same has been reported for some cases of rheumatoid arthritis. The problem, it appears, is not the fat or lactose, at least not for these conditions. The trigger seems to be the dairy proteins.

Dairy products are linked to other health problems ranging from acne to prostate and ovarian cancer. It is the latter issue—cancer—that has gotten the attention of the medical community. Two large Harvard studies and several studies from other countries have shown that milk-drinking men have a significantly higher risk of prostate cancer compared with men who generally avoid dairy products.[13–16] In trying to explain this association, researchers have pointed fingers at milk's hormonal effects, as well as potentially harmful effects of its high calcium and phosphate content.[17] For ovarian cancer, the evidence is mixed, with some studies showing higher risk among milk drinkers and others showing no increased risk.[18, 19, 20]

Milk's selling point has been the calcium it provides. There are, however, better calcium sources and more effective ways of maintaining strong bones. I will go into more detail about this later in the chapter.

Making better choices. People who avoid dairy products find no shortage of great substitutes. Health food stores and regular supermarkets stock soy milk, rice milk, almond milk, and many others. They come in regular, calcium-fortified, and low-fat varieties and in plain vanilla, chocolate, and strawberry flavors. You will want to choose those lowest in fat and sugar. Calcium-fortified juices have arrived on the market, too. Of course, none of these is necessary. After the age of weaning, the only beverage that is actually biologically required is water. Not soda, not juice, not milk—just pure water.

There are many delicious nondairy ice cream substitutes made from soy or rice milk. In many cases, however, the main reason they are so delicious is that they contain added sugar. Your taste buds can be easily seduced by these treats, but your body would be far better off with a bowl of strawberries.

Alternatives to Eggs

There are just two problems with eggs: the yolk and the white. The yolk is where cholesterol lurks, with around 200 milligrams in a single egg. That's similar to an 8-ounce steak.

The yolk also holds the fat, about 5 grams per egg. Egg white has problems of its own, since it is essentially pure animal protein. As you know by now, animal protein can present problems for your kidneys, and you are better off with plant protein.

Can there really be all that fat, cholesterol, and animal protein inside a single egg? Certainly. Keep in mind that when an egg hatches, a baby chick emerges. That chick's body—legs, wings, skin, feathers, internal organs, and everything else—was formed from what was inside the egg when it was laid. So it was loaded with cholesterol and other things you do not want. Like all animal products, eggs have no fiber at all and no complex carbohydrate.

There are plenty of great ways to replace eggs, whether you are hooked on scrambled eggs for breakfast or baked goods that include eggs. Try these substitutes.

- If a recipe calls for just 1 or 2 eggs, leave them out. Add a couple of extra tablespoons of water for moisture.

- Egg replacement powders are available in many health food stores.

- Use 1 heaping tablespoon soy flour or cornstarch plus 2 tablespoons water to replace each egg in baked products.

- Try an egg-size piece of mashed tofu in place of each egg.

- Half a mashed banana can be used in muffin and cookie recipes, although it will provide its own flavor.

- For meatless loaves and veggie burgers, use any of the following to bind the ingredients together: tomato paste, mashed potato, moistened bread crumbs, or rolled oats.

- For a breakfast dish to replace scrambled eggs, scrambled tofu has become popular. Tofu has a texture very much like egg white and takes on the flavor of whatever it is cooked with. Be wary of products promoted as no-cholesterol egg replacements; many are simply egg whites with various added ingredients.

2. KEEP VEGETABLE OILS TO A MINIMUM

Oils creep in everywhere, it seems: cooking oils, salad oils, vegetable oils used in baking and in snack foods. Vegetable oils do enjoy a better reputation than animal fat, and indeed, they have less saturated fat—the kind that raises cholesterol levels. But we still want to keep *all* oils to a minimum. Here is why.

First, as we saw above, all fats and oils are loaded with calories. They have 9 calories per gram, which is more than twice the calorie content of carbohydrate or protein (4 calories per gram). Thus, when it comes to calorie content, vegetable oils are as fattening as lard. All fats and oils are in fact equally fattening.

Second, if your goal is to regain as much insulin sensitivity as possible, you will want to eliminate not only animal fats but also added vegetable oils. Cleaning the animal fat out of your cellular "locks" does no good if you are going to clog them with vegetable grease. Here are the sources of these oils.

Fried foods. French fries, potato chips, onion rings, and other fried snacks are essentially sponges carrying grease from the deep fryer to your body fat stores.

Added oils. Typical salad dressings and margarines have lots of fat.

Oils used as ingredients. Many packaged foods and sauces include significant amounts of oil.

Oils used in sautéing. Many recipes begin with the instruction to sauté onions, garlic, or other ingredients in oil. Some restaurants use oil almost as a staple.

There are easy ways to avoid all that grease.

- Steer clear of fried snacks such as potato chips and french fries.

- Top salads with fat-free dressings, lemon juice, balsamic vinegar, or seasoned rice vinegar.

- Use nonstick pans.

- Steam-fry onions, garlic, or vegetables in water or another cooking liquid instead of sautéing the traditional way.

- Steam vegetables.

- In place of poured oils, consider using cooking spray. If you use just a quick spritz, the amount of added oil is trivial.

- Use fat-free nondairy coffee creamer.

- Read package labels. Look for products with no more than 3 grams of fat per serving or with a percentage of calories from fat of below 10 percent.

When it comes to avoiding greasy foods, some people are eager to make an exception for olive oil. It seems natural and even chic. But think for a second about how factories manage to fill a bottle with oil. They take an enormous number of olives, discard their fiber and pulp, and leave you with the fat.

Gram for gram, olive oil has the same number of calories as beef fat, chicken fat, and other fats and oils—that is, 9 calories per gram. No other food is more calorie dense. While olive oil contains a great deal of monounsaturated fat, which has little or no effect on cholesterol, it also contains saturated fat (about 14 percent), the kind that increases cholesterol and worsens insulin resistance. It does not matter how expensive the oil is or how "extra virgin" it may be. It still has more calories and saturated fat than your body is designed to process to maintain optimal health.

There are, of course, traces of natural vegetable oils in vegetables, fruits, beans, and grains, but you need not worry about them. Your body does need a tiny amount of fat, and plants provide it naturally. We run into problems when oils are concentrated, as they are in fried foods, oily sauces, and recipes with added oils.

A few plant foods, such as nuts, seeds, olives, avocados, and some soy products, are naturally high in oil. If you are trying to lose weight or tackle diabetes, you will want to avoid them.

What about Good Fats?

There are two types of fat your body actually needs. Their technical names are alpha-linolenic acid and linoleic acid. These terms are not important; you will never see them on an ingredients list. What is important to know is that you need only a tiny amount of them. The body's need for these essential fats is no more than 2 to 3 percent of your daily calorie intake.

Where do you find them? Beans, vegetables, and fruits are very low in fat overall, but the traces they do contain are relatively rich in "good" fat—that is, alpha-linolenic acid. This is the basic omega-3 fat that your body uses to produce other good fats. Nuts, seeds, and soy products contain larger amounts. Linoleic acid is found in many plant foods, too.

Some people boost the omega-3 fats in their diets. If you are doing this, be careful: All fats, good and bad, are equally fattening, and many contain things your body does not need. Fish oil, for example, contains plenty of saturated fat along with its omega-3s.

The best way to get the right kind and amount of fat in your diet is to skip animal products, fried foods, and oily food products and get your nutrition from vegetables, fruits, beans, and whole grains.

Does it really matter whether or not we avoid animal products and added oils? Absolutely. A typical North American or European diet might provide 80 to 100 grams of fat per day, or even more. Switching from beef to chicken and fish, keeping portions modest, and limiting added oils will trim this to about 60 grams. But setting animal products aside and avoiding added oils can drop this number to close to 20 grams. In the process, your cholesterol intake, which would be well over 200 milligrams per day on an unmodified diet, will drop to zero. Every cell in your body will thank you.

3. FAVOR FOODS WITH A LOW GLYCEMIC INDEX

You will find this third guideline very useful. The glycemic index (GI) is a handy tool that was invented by David Jenkins, MD, PhD, DSc, a physician and researcher at the University of Toronto.[21] It is simply a number that indicates how rapidly any given food releases sugar into the bloodstream. A food with a high GI releases sugar into the blood quickly.

One example is white bread. If a molecule of carbohydrate in bread was greatly magnified, it would look like a string of beads. Each bead is a molecule of sugar (glucose). In your digestive tract, these beads separate and pass into your bloodstream.

With white bread, this process is quick. The string of beads rapidly disintegrates, and the individual glucose molecules race into your bloodstream. If you were to check your blood sugar after eating the bread, you would see the result. White bread has a high GI, meaning it has a pronounced effect on your blood glucose.

In contrast, pumpernickel bread has a low GI.* Its "beads" come apart more slowly, passing into the bloodstream bit by bit. It has much less effect on your blood sugar.

In a nutshell, high-GI foods tend to have a greater effect on your blood sugar, and low-GI foods have less effect.

I should mention that when researchers measure the GI of individual foods, they test volunteers who do not have diabetes, so a food that does not raise their blood sugar very much could raise yours somewhat more. However, the point of the glycemic index is to allow us to rate foods—to compare one against another—so we can choose the best ones.

If you were to do an online search for information about the Glycemic Index, you would soon discover a mind-numbing array of tables from a variety of sources, none of which agree with each other. That is because the GI of any food can vary depending on the brand, how it was prepared, and other factors. So, let's keep things simple. Here is all you need to know about the GI:

Glycemic Index at a Glance

- White and wheat breads are high GI. Rye and pumpernickel are better choices.

- Table sugar is high GI. Fruits are better. They give you a sweet taste with a suprisingly low GI.

---

*The glycemic index of a food is determined by feeding a portion containing 50 grams of carbohydrate to 10 healthy people after an overnight fast. Blood glucose is tested at 15- to 30-minute intervals over the next 2 hours, and the result is compared to feeding the same amount of glucose (or, in some cases, white bread). A GI below 100 means the food has less effect on blood sugar, compared to glucose. A higher number means the test food has a greater effect.[22]

- White baking potatoes are high GI. Sweet potatoes are lower.

- Most cold cereals are high GI (especially if they have a toy inside the box). Oatmeal and bran cereals are better.

And here are a few more tips, for extra credit:

- Beans and their relatives (lentils, peas) are always low GI.

- Green leafy vegetables can also be considered low GI (although they have so little starch that their GIs typically have not been calculated).

- Pasta is a low-GI food. Because pasta is compacted (unlike bread), it digests slowly and releases its natural sugars only gradually. More on this below.

- Barley, bulgur, and parboiled (converted) rice all have a low GI value.

Now, if you have type 2 diabetes, *any* food with carbohydrate in it will push your blood sugar up to a degree. In fact, a rise in blood glucose after a meal is normal, and if your cells are insulin resistant, it takes a bit more time for glucose in your bloodstream to pass into your cells. This does not mean, however, that you should avoid foods that contain carbohydrate. What it means is that you will want to take steps to reduce your insulin resistance, as outlined in this chapter. Among carbohydrates, the best are those with a low GI.

The reason I mention this is that sometimes people with type 2 diabetes shun carbohydrates. They avoid rice, beans, pasta, and all the rest and load up on chicken, fish, and eggs because these foods have no carbohydrate. But over the long run, they find their blood sugar does not improve; their level gets worse, so they need more and more medicine. It makes sense when you think about the fact that these foods contribute a load of fat and aggravate the accumulation of fat in cells—more gum in the locks, so to speak. Greasy meals today mean insulin resistance tomorrow.

It may surprise you to learn that pasta has a low GI. It does, particularly if it is served *al dente*, that is, not overcooked. Of course, pasta is made from wheat flour, so you may think it would spike your blood sugar in the same way as wheat bread. But that is not the case.

Pasta actually gives us a little lesson in why some foods have a high GI, while the GI of others is low.

Let's say we are making bread dough. We add a bit of yeast to the flour to make the bread rise. The yeast causes many tiny air pockets to form, which is what makes bread different from, say, a shingle. Now, as you eat the baked bread, your stomach acid and digestive enzymes enter those air pockets and rapidly break the molecules of flour into individual sugar molecules that then pass from your digestive tract into your bloodstream. Even whole wheat bread, with shreds of fiber remaining, is easy pickings for digestive enzymes—they have no difficulty entering the air pockets and digesting the starch in the bread.

Pasta is different. It is not made with yeast, so it has no air pockets. If bread is like a pile of tiny twigs, ready to ignite with a single spark, pasta is like a cord of logs—it is much more compacted and "catches fire" more slowly. Even if you chew pasta thoroughly, there is no way it can digest as rapidly as bread—and that's why it has a lower GI.

The take-home lesson is that processing foods—pulverizing grains into flour or using yeast to make dough rise, for example—starts the digestive process before you even put the food on your plate. An intact grain is slow to come apart and release glucose into your bloodstream, while a heavily processed grain is likely to disintegrate quickly. Thus, old-fashioned oatmeal, which consists of whole oats, has a low GI. But quick-cooking oatmeal is made by slicing the oat grains into fragments. That allows it to cook faster and to digest faster—which means a higher GI.

If you would like to look up the GI of individual foods, you can take a look at a Web site established at the University of Sydney in Australia: glycemicindex.com. Just type in the name of the food, and all the testing results will appear.

"Does it really matter?" you may be asking. "Can it really make a difference if my oatmeal is old-fashioned instead of instant, or if I bring beans, green leafy vegetables, and barley soups into my life?" Jennie Brand-Miller, PhD, of the University of Sydney, answered that question by analyzing the combined results of 14 studies on the glycemic index that included a total of 356 participants. She found that choosing low-GI foods reduces hemoglobin A1C by 0.3 to 0.4 percentage point. In some studies, the difference was as much as 0.6 point.[23] Studies showed a similar benefit for both type 1 and type 2 diabetes.

This advantage is over and above that of the other diet changes you are making. As you will remember from Chapter 2, the combined diet changes described in this book—avoiding animal products, minimizing oils, and eating low-GI foods—added up to an A1C drop of 1.2 percentage points, on average, in our research. That average includes people who did not have very far to drop as well as some participants who started with A1Cs in the 9 to 10 percent range and dropped several percentage points. These results are stronger than any single drug is likely to bring. For some people, that is all it takes to return their A1C to the normal range.

TWO IMPORTANT SUPPLEMENTS

Fruits, vegetables, beans, and grains provide the healthy nutrition you need. Eating these foods, you are much better nourished than you would be on a meaty, dairy-filled diet, because these healthy, plant-based foods are rich in fiber, vitamins, and other plant-based nutrients, while helping you skip unhealthful fats and cholesterol. Even so, there are two supplements that are important for you to know about.

Vitamin B$_{12}$. Vitamin B$_{12}$ is essential for healthy nerves and healthy blood cells. If your B$_{12}$ level runs low, you could have nerve symptoms that are permanent. But this vitamin is not made by animals or plants. Rather, it is produced by bacteria. How does this substance get from bacteria to the human body? Some have suggested that before the advent of modern hygiene, there were traces of bacteria in the soil, on vegetables and fruits, on our fingers, or in our mouths that provided the tiny traces of vitamin B$_{12}$ that we need. Whether that was ever true, it is certainly not a reliable source today. Bacteria in animals' intestinal tracts produce vitamin B$_{12}$, and traces of it end up in meat and other animal products. The problem with these sources is that along with it come cholesterol, fat, and animal proteins. B$_{12}$ is also added to some foods, as you will sometimes see on the package labels of breakfast cereals, soymilk, nutritional yeast, and other products. The best source is a vitamin B$_{12}$ supplement, which you will find at any drugstore or health food store, and you should take it daily. The dose is not especially important, because all common brands have more than the recommended daily allowance, and even high doses of B$_{12}$ do not appear to be dangerous.

Vitamin D. Technically, vitamin D is not a vitamin at all. It's actually a hormone produced by sunlight on your skin. Once activated in your liver and kidneys, it helps you absorb calcium and helps protect your cells against cancer, among other functions.

If you get plenty of sun, you do not need any vitamin D in your diet. But if you do not get regular sun exposure, a vitamin D supplement is important. A reasonable daily dose is 2,000 IU.

PUTTING THE RIGHT FUEL IN YOUR TANK

Now we have covered the basics, the three guidelines that work together to help you regain control: avoiding animal products, keeping oils to a minimum, and favoring low-GI foods.

These guidelines work together. Meeting one of them is not enough. For example, jelly beans can be vegan, and they are low in oil. Because they are essentially solid sugar, though, they have a high GI and will spike your blood glucose.

Similarly, a snack cake loaded with butter can have a very low GI because butter contains no carbohydrate and may even slow the absorption of glucose you eat. But the snack cake is not vegan, nor is it low in fat. It will contribute to insulin resistance, and you want to steer clear of it. The low GI is not a reason to eat it if it does not meet our other criteria.

The three guidelines together are a powerful combination. Nancy's A1C was 8.3 percent at the beginning of our study. As she began the healthy diet changes, it rapidly slid under 7.0, even while she reduced her medications. For Vance, initial A1C testing showed a value of 9.5 percent, but as the weeks went by, it dropped and dropped and dropped. By the study's conclusion, his A1C was a healthy 5.3 percent.

Now, before we plan out your breakfast, lunch, and dinner, let me show you how these three principles translate into changes inside your body. Just as a car performs dramatically better when it has the fuel it was designed for, your body performs far better when you give it the foods it needs.

Increased insulin sensitivity. As you know by now, evidence shows that a diet change can have a quick and decisive influence on the amount of fat inside your cells. As the amount of fat drops, your cells become more and more sensitive to insulin, allowing your blood sugar to come down. If your insulin resistance was previously worsening and your medication doses increasing, the process begins to reverse.

This can happen remarkably quickly. In fact, it can happen so quickly that it is essential, if you are using insulin or any drug that increases insulin secretion (for example, glipizide, glimepiride, glyburide, nateglinide, or repaglinide), that you be in close touch with your doctor. As your cells regain their insulin sensitivity, you will become more and more like a healthy person who is taking drugs he or she no longer needs.

The combination of a healthy diet and the drugs you have been taking can drive your blood sugar down to healthful levels and then below them, to hypoglycemia. In other words, your blood sugar can fall too low, which can be dangerous. Your doctor will lower your medication doses or even discontinue your medications as necessary, which will solve the problem. Now, do not throw your medicines away on your own. Your doctor will guide you. And do not be frightened by this return to health. It is a wonderful feeling to discover that your insulin sensitivity is improving day by day. When your doctor says it's time to cut back on medication or stop a drug altogether, it is as if time is moving backward.

Chapter 7 has important details on how to prevent and treat hypoglycemic episodes. Please read it carefully before you change your diet.

Easy weight control. If you have been hoping to lose weight, that process has just begun. On average, the diet you are beginning causes a weight loss of about 1 pound per week. As time goes on, it adds up to an impressive change.

"How does this work?" you may ask. How can you lose weight if you are paying no attention at all to portion sizes, calories, and carbohydrates? There are three main reasons.

First, the foods have very little fat, so you are eliminating the main source of unwanted calories.

Second, the vegetables, fruits, beans, and whole grains you are bringing into your diet give you a healthy dose of fiber, which is filling enough to turn off your appetite a bit sooner than would happen without them. On average, each 14 grams of fiber cuts about 10 percent off your calorie intake. A person who normally eats 2,000 calories per day and then starts to add an extra 14 grams of fiber daily will tend to feel full after eating 1,800 calories.[24]

Third, these foods cause a slight boost in your after-meal calorie burn. Normally, you burn calories faster after a meal due to the processes of digestion. Our studies have shown that a low-fat vegan diet increases this after-meal burn, giving you an extra edge.[25] I will go over this in more detail in Chapter 6. For now, just enjoy the weight control that is kicking in on its own.

Losing excess weight feels great, of course, but weight loss improves your insulin sensitivity in addition to the effects of the diet change itself.

Easy cholesterol control. If you have had a cholesterol problem, the program you are now beginning is far more powerful than typical cholesterol-lowering diets. This should be no surprise. Your new diet is not *low* in cholesterol; it has no cholesterol *at all*. It also has no animal fat, which is important because animal fat (like other sources of saturated fat) encourages your body to make cholesterol. They are all gone now. You have replaced them with cholesterol-lowering oats, soy, and other botanical magicians, as you will see in more detail in Chapter 12.

Your arteries are starting to breathe a sigh of relief. The damage of diabetes is done to the arteries, for the most part, leading to problems in your heart, eyes, kidneys, and nerves. But now, you are inhibiting that process, and bringing your cholesterol level down is part of it. You are following the kind of diet used in programs to *reverse* heart disease.

Again, do not throw your medications away and cancel your doctor appointments. Your doctor can size up your heart health and track your progress.

Reversing symptoms. A team of California researchers used a low-fat vegan diet, combined with exercise, in a group of 21 people with type 2 diabetes, all of whom had painful neuropathy—the nerve symptoms that arise as the nerves are damaged. In just 2 weeks, 17 of the 21 reported complete cessation of their nerve symptoms, and the remaining 4 had noticeable improvements.[26] So our research team did a test of a low-fat, vegan diet alone—without exercise—and found that, indeed, it can improve nerve function and reduce neuropathy symptoms.[27]

Other researchers have found that some of the changes in the eye—exudates in the retina—that sometimes occur in diabetes start to improve or even disappear when people make a healthy diet change. The loss of protein through the kidneys can also diminish. You will find more details on all of these in Chapter 13.

FIRST STEPS

One of the things we have carefully tested with this program is how people *feel* about it. Bottom line: Although you will be making major changes in your menu that are designed to bring you uncompromised good health, this is perhaps the easiest diet change to stick with over the long run. Partly, that is because it is not a "diet." It is a different way of regarding food—a much better way of thinking about and enjoying it. Also, you will never go hungry and never tease yourself with minuscule portions of foods you love.

Let me show you the steps that make it that way. For the moment, you are not actually going to change anything. I just want to walk you through the steps that will get you started.

Step 1: Check Out the Possibilities

Before you jump into a new way of eating, take a week and check out a few recipes and new food products. Look through the next chapter for ideas. You will find a great many possibilities to get you started. If you rarely cook and tend to eat at restaurants, the next chapter will have many tips on things you can look for.

Your goal is to identify healthy breakfasts, lunches, and dinners that you really like. That means meals that meet all of our guidelines (no animal products, minimal vegetable oils, and low GI) *and* appeal to your tastes.

Remember that this new way of eating does not mean making a new dish every night. William Castelli, MD, former director of the Framingham Heart Study, used to say that most of us tend to stick to our favorite meals. We may have four or five different dinners we like, and we pick from that repertoire night after night. All you need to do is to find *healthy* meals that suit your tastes, and you are set. A week is more than enough time to do that.

Step 2: Pick 3 Weeks

Some people like to ease their way gradually into a healthier diet pattern. If you are among that group, go ahead and take your time getting to know healthier foods. But I advise a different approach. Mark a 3-week period on your calendar when you plan to embrace this program. Before you reach your start date, identify meals that fit our criteria and appeal to you. When the start day arrives, commit yourself completely for 21 days.

As I tell our research participants, this is not the time to stick your toe in the swimming pool; it's time to jump in. Really do it. Make it all low-fat vegan, all the time. There are two reasons for this.

First, it gives you fast results. If you have a healthy meal on Monday and another on Saturday, your body will not notice any difference. But if you do it at every meal, gains come quickly. Give yourself a chance to see how it feels to be on as perfect a diet as possible.

The second reason is that a diet change really is like getting into a swimming pool. If you ease your way into the water bit by bit, it is a painful process. But if you plunge in, very soon you see that the water feels fine. Let me explain.

Did you ever switch from whole milk to fat-free milk? If you are like most people, that first glass of fat-free seemed watery and maybe even discolored. After a couple of weeks, though, you became totally used to the lighter taste. Before long, whole milk seemed thick and distasteful.

Now, I am not suggesting that fat-free milk is a health food. As you have seen, there are good reasons to avoid it. But when you lighten your diet, your tastes rapidly change. Very soon, you come to prefer the new, healthier taste.

You will find that your taste buds have a memory of about 3 weeks, and jumping into the diet change allows them to adjust quickly. Instead of pining over the unhealthy foods you have left behind, you will be surprised to find that you miss them very little.

If a 100 percent diet change sounds like a tall order, let me make it a bit more approachable. You do not need to commit to it forever; you just need to give it a try. At this point, there's no need to swear off bacon double cheeseburgers, pledge your loyalty to oatmeal, or make any other daunting promises. Just give it 3 weeks. During that time, really do it 100 percent, and you will get a good sense of what the diet will do while still keeping all your options open.

GET TO KNOW TRANSITION FOODS

Modern technology has brought us plenty of modern annoyances (ringing cell phones, crowded freeways, and junk e-mail), but once in a while, it's actually useful. The food industry has managed to mimic unhealthy foods with more healthful varieties.

The hot dog, long reviled by nutritionists, gained a measure of respectability once food scientists figured out how to transform soybeans into a frankfurter. Veggie hot dogs, veggie burgers, and veggie sausages debuted in health food stores but are now sold everywhere. Even deli salami, turkey, chicken, and bologna slices have soy or wheat counterparts that look and taste very much like the real thing, with zero animal fat and cholesterol.

These foods are hardly the pinnacle of fine dining, but they are practical. If you have children, they are an absolute gift. If you saw what goes into a real hot dog, it would become the last thing you would want to see heading for your child's mouth. But a veggie version is something you can bring home with pride—and your kids will love them. These products help you through the transition to a broader range of healthy foods.

Soy milk has arrived big time. Once, buying soy milk meant shopping at a health food store that was dingy and dark. The cashier was wearing a tie-dyed shirt, his name was Sunshine, and folk music was playing in the background.

Well, those days are gone. Health food stores are big businesses that know a thing or two about customer service. Regular supermarkets stock dozens of flavors of soy milk, along with rice milk, almond milk, oat milk, and other varieties, too, and people from all walks of life enjoy them.

As you shop for meat and dairy substitutes, take a look at the labels. When you check the ingredient lists, you will see that some products are not quite as vegan as you might like because they include egg whites or dairy proteins. Choose the vegan versions, and look for those that are lowest in fat.

COMPLETE NUTRITION

When you follow the nutrition guidelines in this chapter, your diet is likely to improve dramatically.[28] Not only will you skip all the animal fat and cholesterol, you will get much more of the healthy nutrients your body needs: soluble fiber to cut cholesterol, healthy vitamins to reduce cancer risk, potassium to lower blood pressure, and antioxidants to knock out free radicals, to name a few.

Even so, you are making a big change, and you are likely to wonder whether you are missing out on anything. Let me offer a word of reassurance. If you choose your meals from a variety of whole grains, legumes, vegetables, and fruits and take my advice about vitamin B_{12} and vitamin D, above, you will have your bases covered.

Here's where the healthy nutrients are on your plate.

Protein. Your body uses protein to build and repair body tissues. Proteins are made up of small molecules called amino acids. All the proteins in your skin, muscles, bones, and internal organs are built from various combinations of about 20 different amino acids.

A healthy diet of beans, grains, vegetables, and fruits provides all the protein you need. In fact, you are better off getting protein from plant sources. While animal protein can be hard on the delicate tissues of the kidneys, plant proteins appear to be free of this problem. They are also free of the risks of calcium loss and kidney stones associated with animal protein.[29] Animal protein tends to cause calcium to pass through the kidneys and into the urine. In the process, calcium is not only lost, but it ends up in your urinary tract, where it can cause stones.

In years past, some nutritionists believed that vegetarians needed to carefully combine various foods in order to get adequate protein. The idea was that foods from plants might be missing one or more amino acids, so only combining foods in certain ways could ensure that you got them all. This notion was set aside long ago. The Academy of Nutrition and Dietetics' official position statements make it clear that plant-based diets provide plenty of protein without combining foods in any particular way.[30] If, for any reason, you wish to increase your protein intake, turn to the bean group. You will find extra amounts of protein in soy products, such as tofu, tempeh, and soy milk, and in wheat derivatives (e.g., seitan) used to make meat substitutes.

Calcium. For many people, calcium and milk are almost synonymous. They think that milk will build strong bones and protect against fractures later in life. Research has shown, however, that milk's benefits are, for the most part, a myth. Studies do not show much benefit for the bones from drinking milk. How can that be? Well, only about one-third of milk's calcium is absorbed by the body. The other two-thirds simply passes out with the wastes. In addition, milk contains animal protein and sodium, both of which tend to increase calcium loss through the kidneys.

Do not misunderstand me here—you need some calcium in your diet, but it should come from healthful sources, namely green leafy vegetables and beans. While there is somewhat less calcium in broccoli than in milk, the absorption fraction—the percentage that your body can actually use—is higher for broccoli and nearly all other greens than for milk. There is one exception: Spinach is high in calcium, but the absorption fraction is very low.

Greens and beans will give you the calcium your body needs. If you are looking for extra calcium for whatever reason, you can find plenty more in fortified juices and soy milks.

To maintain calcium balance, however, it is important not only to take in an adequate amount but also to minimize losses. Animal protein causes your body to lose calcium through the kidneys, and it can be measured in the urine. Studies of high-protein diets, such as the Atkins Diet, dramatically demonstrate the losses: Such diets increased calcium loss by more than 50 percent.[31] It is also important to limit sodium (salt) and get vitamin D from either sunlight or supplements. Vegetables and fruits promote bone strength for reasons that are not entirely clear, and exercise gives your bones a reason to live. It is a strong determiner of bone health. Finally, it is also important to avoid tobacco, since smoking increases fracture risk.

Iron. Iron is a double-edged sword. You need iron to build hemoglobin, which your red blood cells use to carry oxygen from your lungs to your body tissues. But too much iron can be toxic. It can increase the risk of heart problems and may even worsen insulin resistance.

Iron encourages the production of unstable molecules called free radicals, which can damage your body's delicate tissues and are linked to heart disease, cancer, and even certain aspects of the aging process.

The most healthful iron sources are the same foods that bring you calcium: beans and green leafy vegetables. They are rich in iron but carry it in a special form called non-heme iron. Your body easily absorbs this form when it's in need of more iron, but the iron passes harmlessly out of the body when you have all you need. In contrast, meats contain heme iron, which is like an uninvited guest at your party: It barges in whether you need it or not. Over the long run, meat eaters tend to accumulate too much iron.

If you are anemic, do not rush out and buy iron supplements, or worse, add lots of meat to your diet. Instead, work with your doctor to find out what kind of anemia you have and *why* it occurred. Anemia can be a sign of kidney disease; it can be caused by certain drugs; and it can be a sign of blood loss from your digestive tract caused by gastrointestinal irritation or even colon cancer. It is essential that you be evaluated and treated appropriately.

If you do need extra iron, turn first to greens and beans. Vitamin C–rich foods, such as fruits and vegetables, increase the absorption of iron from the other foods you eat, and avoiding dairy products helps, too. They are very low in iron and actually reduce its absorption from your digestive tract.

Zinc. Zinc plays important roles in immune function, wound healing, and many other biological functions, but as with iron, you can have too much of a good thing. The most healthful sources include legumes, nuts, and fortified breakfast cereals (e.g., Post Grape-Nuts, bran flakes, and granola).

Fat. Good fats, bad fats, and too much fat—how do we make sense of it all? The most important fat fact is this: Your body's actual fat requirement is minuscule, as you saw earlier. Most people in Western countries get many times the needed amount. With meats and dairy products front and center in their diets, they not only get too much fat overall, they also get the wrong kind—*saturated* fat, which boosts cholesterol and aggravates insulin resistance.

Nuts, seeds, avocados, olives, and full-fat soy products are also high in fat. Although they are low in saturated fat, the overall amount is high, and you should limit these foods accordingly.

As you also saw earlier, most vegetables, fruits, and beans contain very little fat, and what they do have is a healthful mixture, including traces of the essential fats alpha-linolenic acid and linoleic acid.

If, for any medical reason, you are increasing your oil intake, healthful sources of omega-3 fats include walnuts, soy products, flaxseed, and, in concentrated form, flax, linseed, canola, and walnut oils. Health food stores even sell omega-3 supplements (e.g., DHA) drawn entirely from botanical sources. They are a better choice than fish oils. Omega-6 oils are also sometimes used for health conditions such as arthritis, usually in the form of evening primrose oil, borage oil, black currant oil, or hemp oil. They should be thought of as medicinal supplements rather than as foods.

In the next chapter, you will get started with your new program, and then, in Chapter 7, I will show you how to track your progress.

CHAPTER 5

How to Get Started

By now, you understand the principles for building a healthful diet and are ready to get started with foods that will tame your blood sugar, help you lose weight, and go a long way toward lowering your blood pressure and cholesterol. But you are no doubt asking, how do I start? And will it be easy? Will I be able to stick with it?

Let me put your mind at ease. The two-step system described in the last chapter makes this very easy. You just take a week to "check out the possibilities" and then do a 3-week "test drive." Let's revisit this in more detail:

STEP 1: CHECK OUT THE POSSIBILITIES

Take a week, and see which healthy foods you like best. You are not going to eliminate anything. Rather, you'll try out new products, new recipes, and new tastes, and perhaps get reacquainted with a few healthy tastes you may have forgotten.

Take out a sheet of paper and jot down the headings "Breakfast," "Lunch," "Dinner," and "Snacks." Over the next 7 days, write down— in each of the four categories—foods you like that meet the three guidelines set out in the previous chapter. In a nutshell, we are choosing foods that are:

Vegan. They contain no animal products. This means no meat, fish, dairy products, or eggs—not even a little bit. The idea is to clean the animal fat, animal protein, and cholesterol out of your diet. If you skipped to this chapter and are wondering why these steps are important, please go back and read the preceding chapter.

Low fat. You will use little or no added oil and omit other fatty ingredients. If you are reading labels, choose foods with no more than 3 grams of fat per serving.

Low glycemic index. You will favor low-GI foods. This means generally avoiding sugar, white bread products, baking potatoes, most cold cereals, and a few other foods. Most other vegan foods are fine. Certain foods have an especially low GI value: beans and other legumes, green leafy vegetables, most fruits, barley (which is great in soups), and the many foods that are made from them. Surprisingly, pasta has a low glycemic index, unlike other wheat products.

Healthful Breakfast Ideas

Under "Breakfast," your list may well be similar to what you are eating already. Here are a few suggestions.

- Hot cereals such as oatmeal or other whole grain cereal with cinnamon, raisins, and/or applesauce (no milk)
- Cold cereals such as bran flakes with fat-free soy or rice milk and/or berries, peaches, or bananas
- Melon, cantaloupe, bananas, or any other fruit
- Rye or pumpernickel toast topped with cinnamon (no butter or margarine)

If you like extra protein, try these.

- Veggie sausage
- Veggie bacon
- Scrambled tofu
- Breakfast burritos filled with "refried" beans, lettuce, and tomato (no egg or cheese)
- English baked beans or chickpeas
- Pumpernickel bread with hummus

Here are a few thoughts about some good breakfast choices.

Oatmeal. Most of our research participants make old-fashioned oatmeal a part of their morning routine, and for good reason. Oats are rich in *soluble* fiber—the kind that gets creamy in water and removes cholesterol from your body. (Wheat and rice are high in *insoluble* fiber.) But that humble bowl of oatmeal does more than that. It helps bring your blood sugar under control, and its high fiber content helps you lose weight.

An additional advantage comes from what oats *do not* have: cholesterol and animal fat. A bacon-and-eggs breakfast has a strikingly large amount of both.

Generally speaking, old-fashioned oatmeal is better than instant or 1-minute varieties, although even these quick-cooking versions are far better than bacon and eggs. The more intact the grain, the lower the GI, and the longer the cereal keeps you satisfied. See page 86 for tips on making the perfect bowl of hot oatmeal.

For an extra blood sugar–lowering effect, top your bowl with cinnamon (see page 145 for details about how cinnamon affects blood sugar). Or add raisins, berries, or just about any fruit or mix of fruits you like, but set the milk and sugar aside. Within just a day or two, you will break the habit of adding these unnecessary and unhealthful toppings. If you just cannot imagine oatmeal without milk, splash on some soy milk or rice milk; you will skip the animal fat and cholesterol of cow's milk.

Most dry cereals have a high GI, but oatmeal is in a good GI range, as is bran cereal. They will keep you full and satisfied and help keep your blood sugar steady.

Veggie sausage or bacon. Regular sausage and bacon are loaded with cholesterol and fat and are among the most unhealthful foods on anyone's grocery list. But if you are unable to imagine breakfast without these meats, food manufacturers have come to your rescue with vegan versions, and most supermarkets and all health food stores now carry several varieties. If they are new to you, think of them as a liberal interpretation of the original; they are tasty and high in protein. Read the package labels, and choose those that omit animal ingredients (some are made with egg white, which is concentrated animal protein that you want to avoid) and are as low in fat as possible.

Scrambled tofu. Tofu is almost identical to egg white—it has little flavor of its own but quickly takes on the flavors of whatever spices or sauces it is cooked with. Scrambled tofu is a great substitute for scrambled eggs—it has all the taste but no cholesterol, animal fat, or animal protein. Supermarkets sell scrambled tofu seasoning mixes, usually shelved near boxed rices or in the health food section. Just follow the package directions.

Breakfast burritos. No time for breakfast? Breakfast burritos to the rescue. You buy them frozen, pop them in the microwave, and in a couple of minutes, you have a hearty, healthy breakfast. Health food stores and most regular grocery stores stock a variety of frozen burritos made with beans, tofu, tomatoes, and other ingredients. You can also make your own, of course, perhaps on the weekend, and refrigerate or freeze them so they are handy for those busy mornings.

Bagels. If bagels are your thing, favor pumpernickel bagels, which have a lower GI than white bagels.

A Few Things Not on the Breakfast Menu

Just to state the obvious, eggs are off the list. A single egg has around 200 milligrams of cholesterol—similar to an 8-ounce steak—plus a load of saturated fat, the kind that tends to raise cholesterol. The white of the egg presents a big dose of animal protein that you want to avoid. As you know, getting your protein from plant sources is better for your kidneys and your long-term bone health. Skip eggs and egg replacements such as Egg Beaters, which are made from egg whites.

Of course, breakfast meats are off the list, too, including turkey sausage as well as pork or beef varieties. They *all* have cholesterol and animal protein.

Forget doughnuts, Danishes, and muffins. To see why, set one on a napkin for a few minutes, then look at how much grease has leached out. That grease is just waiting to fatten you up, boost your cholesterol, and worsen your insulin resistance.

A Balanced Breakfast

You may wish to start your breakfast with a high-protein food such as veggie sausage and follow it with a starchier food like oatmeal with cinnamon and raisins or a sweet food such as fruit. It's not that you need extra protein; there is actually plenty of protein in any typical meal built from vegetables, grains, and beans. Here's why starting with a high-protein food can be helpful.

Starchy or sugary foods naturally increase the production of serotonin—the same feel-good chemical that is boosted by antidepressants such as fluoxetine (Prozac) and sertraline (Zoloft)—in the brain. Now, that's a nice benefit, but for some people, the result is postbreakfast drowsiness. In fact, some people actually use starchy foods as a remedy for insomnia. A high-protein food blocks the serotonin-producing action,

Sample 1-Day Menu

Breakfast

Veggie sausage

Rye toast

Oatmeal with cinnamon and raisins

Sliced cantaloupe

Lunch

Green salad

Split pea soup

Hummus sandwich on rye bread with sliced tomato and cucumber

Dinner

Spinach salad with cherry tomatoes

Angel hair pasta with tomato and mushroom sauce

Steamed broccoli

Snacks

Apples, oranges, bananas

boosting your energy. Any high-protein food will do: veggie sausage, veggie bacon, scrambled tofu, beans, or even a spoonful or two of chickpeas—the kind you'd normally throw on a salad.

So, during this first week, explore the various breakfast possibilities and jot down your favorites.

Healthful Lunch Ideas

Okay, let's move on to lunch. Here are a few ideas, but you will no doubt have many more.

Salads

- Garden salad with fat-free dressing, lemon juice, or soy or teriyaki sauce

- Three-bean salad

- Pasta salad

- Black bean and corn salad

- Grain-based salad, such as noodles, couscous, bulgur, or rice

Soups

- Minestrone

- Mixed vegetable

- Lentil

- Mushroom barley

- Black bean

- Vegetarian chili

- Split pea

- Instant and prepared soups are okay as long as they are low-fat and free of animal products.

Sandwiches/Wraps

- CLT: sliced cucumber, lettuce, and sliced tomato on rye bread with Dijon mustard. Or use veggie bacon, rather than cucumber, if you like.

- Hummus on a whole wheat pita with grated carrots, sprouts, and sliced cucumber

- Sandwich made with fat-free meat alternatives such as veggie turkey, bologna, or pepperoni slices or barbecued seitan (wheat gluten), plus your favorite sandwich veggies on rye bread

- Black bean dip, bell pepper and tomato slices, and lettuce wrapped in a whole wheat tortilla

- Italian eggplant sub: baked eggplant slices, pizza sauce, and mushrooms on a whole grain sub roll

- Black bean and sweet potato burrito with corn and tomatoes

Extras

- Fresh fruit

- Chickpeas

- Cut-up vegetables

Here are a few more details on good lunch choices.

Salads. Salads vary from the simple lettuce-and-tomato variety to pasta salads, three-bean salads, Asian salads, fruit salads, and many others.

If you start with salad greens, regular lettuce is fine, but do not shy away from baby spinach, arugula, and other greens. Add cucumber, artichoke hearts, and tomato slices and by all means, chickpeas, kidney beans, or other legumes to your salad. They provide plenty of nutrition and are great at holding your blood sugar steady.

For convenience, supermarkets carry commercial three-bean and four-bean salads in jars, which are ready when you are. Many stores also have well-stocked salad bars.

When you choose dressings, look for fat-free vegan varieties, which are easy to find at many supermarkets.

Soups. Soup is a great lunch starter, or a big bowl of hearty soup can *be* your lunch. Loaded with vegetables, beans, lentils, barley or other grains, and wonderful flavors, soups are satisfying and wonderfully healthful. If you cook up a big pot on the weekend, you will be ready for the week ahead.

If you are looking for convenience, Manischewitz brand dried soup mixes are time-savers. Just add them to boiling water and let them simmer. If you like, add tomatoes, green chiles, or any frozen or fresh vegetables. Stir a tablespoon or two of nutritional yeast into each bowl for a savory touch. If you add extra carrots, tomatoes, frozen vegetables (e.g., broccoli, kale, cauliflower, or green beans), and spices, you will turn your soup into a stew.

If you'd like to let someone else do the cooking, your supermarket has an endless variety of canned and frozen soups. You need to be selective, but you will find plenty that meet our requirements. Lentil, minestrone, and vegetarian vegetable are good choices. Tabatchnick frozen soups offer generous servings of split pea, mushroom barley, and other flavors with simple ingredients and virtually no fat.

Instant soup comes in a cup and just needs hot water. You might keep a few cups in your desk drawer for emergencies.

To have homemade soup anywhere, pick up an insulated bottle, such as a Thermos, so you can just fill it with soup and take it to work. Your co-workers will wish they had done the same.

One caveat about prepared soups: Some manufacturers overdo it with salt, so it pays to choose lower-sodium brands. Aim to keep your total daily sodium intake to less than 1,500 milligrams.

Sandwiches. Sandwiches are quick and portable, and with the enormous variety of ingredients available these days, they can be healthful, too.

Start with a lower-GI bread, such as rye or pumpernickel. Try any or all of the following fillings.

Hummus is a Middle Eastern dish that has become popular in North America. It is made from chickpeas and spices and has a texture vaguely reminiscent of peanut butter but a milder flavor. Unfortunately, many commercial brands are too high in fat, but who needs them? With a food processor, it takes only about 5 minutes to make your own, and a big batch will last for days.

Meatless deli slices have all the taste of bologna, sliced turkey, or ham with none of the animal fat or cholesterol. They are sold at all health food stores and many supermarkets, and they make great sandwiches. You can find them next to the vegetarian hot dogs, which are also great choices. As always, choose lower-fat brands.

Veggie burgers are easy to make, and commercial brands are widely sold in stores and restaurants. Try a few different brands, and find your favorites. Favor those that are lowest in fat.

A BLT made with veggie bacon, lettuce, tomato, and mustard is a great choice. My own keep-it-simple sandwich is a CLT, made on toasted rye bread with lettuce, sliced cucumber and tomato, sometimes a vegan deli slice or two, and topped with Dijon mustard.

Speaking of condiments, mustard is fat-free; make it your spread of choice. Most mayonnaise spreads are just the opposite—they are loaded with fat. There are now many vegan mayos on the market, but they are not necessarily low in fat. Check the labels.

Frozen meals. The TV dinner has grown up. The amazing variety of frozen foods, plus the convenience of microwave ovens, makes it easy to eat healthful, tasty foods. Some favorites include vegan enchilada or burrito dinners and pizza or pasta dishes.

If lunch means dining out—or perhaps fast food—see Chapter 8 for healthful restaurant choices.

Healthful Dinner Ideas

There is a limitless array of healthful foods for dinner, whether you like to cook or not. Many people enjoy cooking, but many others feel too busy or just cannot be bothered; they tend to choose simple and convenient foods or eat out. Personally, I fall squarely into the second group.

The good news is that both temperaments do very well in this program. Here are a few ideas for starters.

- Pasta marinara: Many commercial sauces are fine. Choose those lowest in fat and free of cheese and other animal products. Add some mushrooms, artichoke hearts, or broccoli or spinach (prepared fresh or frozen), and you will be set.

- Beans and rice: Try Cuban black beans with salsa, vegetarian baked beans, or "refried" beans.

- Soft tacos: Start with a whole wheat tortilla and add beans, lettuce, tomato, and salsa.

- Chili: Vegetarian boxed versions are fine.

- Veggie lasagna: Use low-fat tofu to replace the ricotta, and add layers of grilled veggies.

- Rice pilaf, Spanish rice, or packaged rice dinners: Many commercial brands are fine, but omit the butter.

- Fried rice and vegetables: Use a nonstick pan and season this meal with low-sodium soy sauce.

- Fat-free veggie burgers: Read the labels and choose those lowest in fat and free of cheese and other animal products.

- Fajitas: Lightly sauté sliced bell peppers, onion, and eggplant in a nonstick pan and add fajita seasonings.

- Stew made with chunky vegetables in a savory sauce

- Mushroom stroganoff

Our job for now is not to make you into a chef, but simply to make a realistic 1-day menu of foods you really will eat and enjoy.

It pays to think "international." Many cuisines from around the world have great choices, whether you make them yourself, have them at restaurants, or buy them frozen: Mexican bean burritos, Italian pastas and bean soups, Chinese vegetable and rice dishes, Japanese vegetable sushi with miso soup and salads, Indian curries, Thai dishes, Ethiopian cuisine, and many others. These foods take advantage of the rich tradition of plant-based diets in many countries.

If your idea of dinner is sending out for pizza, it can still be vegan and low in fat. Just ask for all-vegetable toppings, such as mushrooms,

A Balanced Dinner

A good way to make sure your dinner is well balanced is to fill about a quarter of your plate with a legume dish. That means beans, peas, or lentils. So you might choose baked beans, a bean burrito, or black-eyed peas, for example. These foods are rich in protein, soluble fiber, and minerals and have wonderfully low GIs.

Next, fill another quarter of your plate with a starchy food such as brown rice, a yam, or pasta. *Starch* is an unglamorous word, but it really means complex carbohydrate—the healthy, clean-burning fuel that powers your body.

Finally, fill the remaining half of your plate with vegetables. Ideally, choose two different varieties—say, a green vegetable like broccoli and an orange vegetable like carrots. These foods are your nutrition powerhouses. Add fruit for dessert, and you will be set.

You can vary these proportions if you like. As long as your plate is vegan, low fat, and low GI, you will be fine.

There are a million ways to do this. Some people like an Italian or Mediterranean meal, which might include bean soup and pasta with a chunky vegetable sauce. Others prefer Latin American meals, with beans, rice, and vegetables. Some might favor an Asian dinner, with tofu (which counts as a legume because it is made from soybeans), rice, and vegetables. An Indian-inspired plate might include a lentil curry with rice and vegetables.

For Americans from Southern states, many traditional foods fit the bill beautifully: beans or black-eyed peas, rice, and greens (without the traditional fatback).

When my North Dakota parents decided to improve their own way of eating, we substituted a bean dish and vegetable cutlets for the usual meat dish and added yams or sweet potatoes, along with a couple of vegetable choices. Dessert was pears, strawberries, or oranges. See the pattern? It's still there: a bean dish, a starchy food for healthy carbs, vegetables, and fruit for dessert.

peppers, onions, sun-dried tomatoes, and capers. Hold the cheese and ask for extra tomato sauce instead. If you are making pizza at home, you can add veggie pepperoni or other deli slices if you like. For a cheesy taste, sprinkle on some nutritional yeast.

Simple Snack Ideas

Okay, your day's menu is nearly complete. But even if you feel you will not be hungry between meals, pencil in a few snack ideas so you will be ready in case the munchies do hit. A 3:00 p.m. hunger pang can erode your resolve, so stock up on things that you can feel good about eating. Here are some snack suggestions.

Fruits have a surprisingly low GI in most cases, and they are unbeatable for nutritional value. Keep apples, oranges, pears, bananas, and other fruits on hand. Some people like to keep a bowl of cantaloupe and melon chunks in the refrigerator for an instant snack that's ready when they get home. Don't forget tropical favorites, like mangoes and papayas. Dried fruits are acceptable. Surprisingly, their GIs are not necessarily higher than those of fresh fruit. Because their water has been removed, however, it is easy to take in far more calories with dried fruit than with fresh fruit, so it pays to favor the fresh varieties.

Instant soups are great to keep in your desk drawer; just add hot water when you are ready to eat. Minestrone, split pea, lentil, and other varieties are typically vegan and low in fat.

A simple CLT—the sandwich of lettuce and sliced cucumber and tomato with mustard on rye bread I mentioned above—will fill you up, with nothing to regret.

Three-bean salad will hold you until dinner.

Air-popped popcorn skips the fat of the usual kind. Top it with garlic salt, mixed seasonings (e.g., Spike), or nutritional yeast.

Hummus on a whole wheat pita is filling and low in fat if you make it without added oil.

Other simple snacks include bran cereal with soy milk, pumpernickel or rye toast with jam, carrot sticks, and rice cakes (look for simple, unsugared varieties).

STEP 2: A 3-WEEK TEST DRIVE

All right, you are doing great! You have made good choices that will give you a healthy start. Now, let's take a 3-week period and, during that time, let's make it all vegan all the time. That means no animal products at all, keep the oils low, and favor healthy, low-GI foods. At this point, that will be easy, because you picked out the foods you like during week one. No need to whip up something new every day. It is fine to repeat items, use leftovers, or make your life easy in any way you can. Remember, though, do not limit calories or skip meals.

It is essential to be realistic. If you do not enjoy cooking now, that is unlikely to change. Plan to have foods on hand that require little preparation.

Will you be at work? Traveling? Planning ahead is essential. If there is nothing healthful in the company canteen, you will want to pack a lunch. Sometimes when a colleague asks what I am having for lunch, I answer, "*les restes d'hier*." This sounds exotic until I explain that the phrase is actually French for "leftovers." But the fact is, my leftovers sometimes *are* exotic, depending on which restaurant filled the doggie bag!

Let's Go Shopping

It pays to stock your shelves with the foods and ingredients you will need so your 3-week test drive goes smoothly. And when hunger hits, you will be ready.

Take a trip down those aisles at the supermarket that you may well have neglected in the past. The produce department may stock meat substitutes, soy milk, and other healthy products, along with an ever-growing array of new and interesting fruits and vegetables. Also check out the "international," "health," and "dietetic" aisles. And look at the shelves with innumerable varieties of rice and colorful dried beans.

Be sure to check out your nearest health food store if you have not done so already. You will find substitutes for meat and milk and interesting foods from other countries, all worth a try. Explore and experiment; some new finds will become favorites. If the occasional purchase turns out to be a dud, do not worry. That is what experimenting is all about.

As you shop, pick up ingredients that will allow you to prepare a few extra things on the weekend—a pot of soup or stew, for example—that you can then split into portions for quick reheating during the week.

You will notice that prices for healthful foods vary widely. Overall, plant-based foods are less expensive than meaty or cheesy products. Beans, fresh and frozen vegetables, pasta, rice—these humble ingredients cost very little. However, health food stores sometimes put premium prices on prepared products, which is true for nonvegetarian as well as healthful vegan items. You will soon sort out your best choices.

While you are at the store, pick up a vitamin B_{12} supplement, and if you do not get regular sunshine, purchase a vitamin D supplement, too.

Some Staples: Basic Foods to Taste and Try

There are a few basic foods that would be good for you to get to know. They are not elaborate—just simple, basic staples that ought to be on your shelves. If they are new to you, they will be healthful additions to your repertoire. Let me list some here and encourage you to think about them when shopping.

Old-fashioned oatmeal. Choose this variety rather than instant, and see how easy and fast it is to make. Just combine 1 part oatmeal with 2 parts cold water, bring to a boil, and simmer for a few minutes. That's all there is to it. Oatmeal is loaded with soluble fiber to bring your cholesterol down and filling enough to keep hunger at bay all morning. While you are at the store, pick up some toppings: cinnamon, raisins or other fruit, or whatever calls to you.

Beans. Get to know the many varieties of this humble food. Very low in fat; devoid of cholesterol; high in soluble fiber, calcium, and iron; and with an enviable glycemic index, beans' day has arrived. Cook them up from scratch if you like, but it's handy to stock your shelves with a couple of cans of black beans (and a jar of salsa), fat-free "refried" beans, and any other varieties you see.

Frozen vegetables. *Convenience* is the word here. If you are the slightest bit pressed for time, you will be glad you have vegetables in your freezer that just need a little steaming. Nutritionally, frozen vegetables are equivalent to fresh. Look for broccoli, winter squash, petite Brussels sprouts, carrots, cauliflower, and anything else you fancy.

Lentil soup. Lentils assert themselves in a hearty and healthful soup. Keep a can or two on hand.

Hummus. As I mentioned above, this simple chickpea dip has become an enormously popular sandwich filling. But skip the commercial brands, which are too high in fat. If you have a food processor, you can make your own in less than 5 minutes, and you will be set for the week.

Chickpeas. Speaking of chickpeas, this is one legume that is really at home just about anywhere—not just as hummus but also in salads, soups, pasta sauces, and stir-fries. You can even eat them for breakfast. Keep a few cans on your shelf; the extra-small cans with pop-top lids are especially convenient.

Toppings. Dijon mustard is great for sandwiches, and lemon juice or apple cider vinegar is great on green vegetables and salads. Salsa was just made for beans, and fat-free dressings of any variety are handy, too.

Brown rice. Most people have never tasted a properly prepared bowl of rice. The trick is to select brown rice, toast it slightly, and cook it like pasta, using what may seem like too much water and draining away the excess at the end.

Barley. This grain is all over the breakfast cereal aisle, in puffed and sugared form, but barley really shines in soups or when served as a grain side dish. You can mix it with rice and cook them together. Barley has a low GI, lots of soluble fiber, and wonderful taste and texture.

Spaghetti sauce. Take a few minutes to read labels on jars of marinara sauce to find varieties that exclude cheese and other animal products and keep oil to a minimum. Then stock your shelves for a quick and easy dinner. Pick up your favorite pasta to go with it.

Meat substitutes. Try the veggie versions of hot dogs, burgers, and deli slices. They are not haute cuisine, but they serve a useful purpose, and some taste surprisingly similar to the foods they imitate. Read the labels, though, and skip products with animal-derived ingredients or more than 2 to 3 grams of fat per serving. Health food stores have a huge selection, and many regular supermarkets carry them, too.

Nutritional yeast. You can find this in the supplement aisle at health food stores. Nutritional yeast dissolves into spaghetti sauces, stir-fries, casseroles, soups, and lots of other recipes, adding a subtle cheese-like taste. It is not the same as brewer's yeast or baker's yeast,

Check the Label

There are two things you want to look for on product labels. First, check the ingredients list to make sure there are no animal-derived ingredients. Common ones include milk solids, whey, casein (and various casein derivatives, such as sodium caseinate), egg products, and gelatin. Also be on the lookout for partially hydrogenated vegetable oils, which are as bad as saturated fat.

Sometimes people want to make exceptions for foods that *sound* as if they are healthful. Honey, for example, has gotten unjustified good press over the decades. Nutritionally speaking, it is simply sugar, offering you nothing from a health standpoint. Rather like olive oil, its marketing has gotten way ahead of its value.

Next, check the Nutrition Facts. Ideally, a serving of food will have no more than about 3 grams of fat and should have zero cholesterol. If the cholesterol content is anything other than zero, the product contains some animal-derived ingredient. If label reading seems a bit cumbersome, keep in mind that you need to check a product only once. As you find the products that fit the bill, there's no need to check them again. Also, simple foods do not need labels. No one ever had to look for the fine print on a banana or pear, a box of frozen spinach, or a bag of navy beans. Each of these foods has exactly one ingredient.

both of which taste bitter. Nutritional yeast comes in flakes and powder. For better texture and versatility, buy the flakes.

Fresh fruit. Fresh fruit is a perfect snack, and you will want to keep it on hand. Buy extra for friends and family.

What to Do with Unhealthy Foods?

So you have filled your shelves and refrigerator with healthy staples. If some not-so-healthful items from your previous diet are still lurking, though, what do you do? That's easy: Get rid of them. Do not "use them up" because they will continue to cause problems for you. Toss them. And if family members or roommates share your kitchen space, avoid keeping tempting foods too near your own. They will present more of a temptation than you need.

Planning Ahead

Eventually, healthful eating will become second nature. For now, though, you will need to put a bit of thought into where you will be at lunchtime and dinnertime and what you will have. There really are healthy choices out there, but they are sometimes not so obvious in a culture that caters to unhealthy tastes. It helps to plan ahead.

ON YOUR MARK, GET SET . . .

As we've discussed, you will want to pick out a 3-week period and really dive into this new menu. Choose a time when you have the mental energy to embrace a change. If you are an accountant, April 14 probably is not a good time. If you are a student, exam week may not be the best choice. But once you have picked your time, jump in with both feet. Do the diet change 100 percent. Follow our three guidelines as closely as humanly possible, and do it all the way.

Okay, you have done great. You have the basics down. In the next several chapters, we will look at specific health issues and situations you may encounter, and I will offer plenty of tips for handling them.

CHAPTER 6

Healthful Weight Control

If you have been aiming to lose weight, let me show you the steps that make the process as easy, effective, and permanent as possible. Eliminating unwanted pounds is important for anyone—but especially for people with diabetes. For starters, it boosts your insulin sensitivity; the more body fat you trim away, the more responsive your cells are to whatever insulin your pancreas is producing.

Weight loss also brings down your cholesterol and blood pressure. And when you've trimmed away body fat, exercise is that much easier and more inviting. Your joints—especially your knees—will thank you.

Needless to say, there are a great many ways to lose weight. Cutting calories works for some people, but others find it a real challenge. If you normally eat 2,000 calories per day, for example, a common recommendation would limit you to 1,500—and that gets old very fast. If you're hungry at 8:00 in the evening and you've already had your 1,500 calories for the day, you will go to bed hungry. That will never happen on the program recommended in this book.

A healthy approach to weight loss focuses on choosing the right kinds of foods, not on the *quantity* of food you eat. When you have the right foods on your side, the calories and portions fall into line on their own, and weight loss is almost automatic.

A WEIGHT-LOSS DIET THAT WORKS

In 2005, my research team published the results of an important study that tested a new and powerful approach to weight loss. The participants were women with moderate to severe weight problems. Most had tried many different diets: low-calorie diets, low-carb diets, Weight Watchers, the cabbage-soup diet, and just about everything else. Like most people, they had found these diets tough to follow, and whatever weight they lost soon returned.

Our approach was very different. It did not include calorie counting, limits on portions or carbohydrates, or even an exercise prescription. For research purposes, we wanted to isolate the effects of diet.

The participants lost weight easily, averaging about 1 pound per week—week after week after week—and they kept it off long-term.[1] Other researchers have found much the same thing.

Why is a plant-based diet so powerful for weight control? Well, first of all, it is important to understand where the calories are hiding in the foods you eat. A chicken stores extra calories in chicken fat. A cow stores calories in beef fat. A fish stores them in fish fat. Body fat—in humans or animals—is a calorie-storage system.

If you were to remove a bit of fat from a drumstick or chicken wing and send it to a laboratory, you would find that a gram of fat— that's $\frac{1}{28}$ ounce—has 9 calories. That is a lot. It is more than double the calories in a gram of carbohydrate—the starch in rice, beans, or sweet potatoes, for example. Carbohydrates have only 4 calories per gram. Small wonder that people who make rice or other plant foods their staples tend to stay slim. Throughout Asia and rural Africa, rice and other grains, root vegetables, and various legumes are the traditional foundation of the diet. These foods are filling but have relatively few calories.

Of course, it's a different story in North America and Europe, where meals feature meat and dairy products, which contain the very fat that animals have used to store their excess calories. Weight problems are the all-too-common result. If you want to avoid taking in extra calories, you would do well to avoid eating the concentrated calories that animals have hidden away in their body fat.

So, step one is to avoid animal products. If you do that, you will of course avoid animal fat completely.

Step two is to keep vegetable oils to a minimum. Beans, grains, vegetables, fruits, and most other foods from plants have very little fat. There are a few exceptions, however: nuts, seeds, avocados, and some soy products are high in fat. Keep them to a minimum as well.

Be especially careful about vegetable oils used in cooking or in salad dressings. Now, some people argue that plant oils are more healthful than animal fats, and it's true that they are much lower in *saturated* fat, the kind that raises cholesterol levels and is linked to breast cancer and insulin resistance. When it comes to weight problems, however, animal fats and vegetable oils are essentially all the same. They all pack in 9 calories per gram.

Step three is to focus on high-fiber foods. A grain of brown rice, for example, has a thin cloak of fiber that gives the rice its tan color. To produce white rice, manufacturers strip away this coating, but you are better off if it is left intact. Fiber fills you up so you feel naturally satisfied with fewer calories.

Steps to Weight Loss

1. Avoid animal products. If you steer clear of fish, chicken, beef, dairy foods, and all other animal products, you will cut your animal fat intake to zero. What's more, this shift will mean that you will naturally eat high-fiber foods to replace those from animal sources, which have no fiber.

2. Keep vegetable oils to a minimum. If you have a bottle of cooking oil in your kitchen, throw it away. There are simpler and better ways to cook. Also limit nuts, seeds, avocados, and full-fat soy products.

3. Favor high-fiber foods. Build your meals from beans and other legumes, vegetables, fruits, and whole grains.

To ensure complete nutrition, be sure to have a vitamin B_{12} supplement each day.

As you saw in Chapter 4, every 14 grams of fiber added to your daily menu cuts calorie intake by about 10 percent on average.[2] That simply means that high-fiber foods fill you up faster, so you stop eating sooner. Instead of trying by sheer force of willpower to cut calories, you cut them *without even thinking about it.*

The richest sources of fiber are beans, vegetables, fruits, and whole grains. While breakfast cereal commercials tend to push grains as the best fiber source, you will find much more fiber in beans and most vegetables than in most grains. But they all add up. Aim for at least 40 grams per day. One caveat: If high-fiber foods, especially beans, have not been part of your routine, you'll want to increase the amount you eat gradually to give your digestive tract time to adjust. See Chapter 9 for more tips on avoiding digestive problems.

In the next chapter, I will show you an easy way to check your fiber intake using the Quick Fiber Check.

Okay, let's summarize: To lose weight, you want to avoid animal products, limit the use of vegetable oils, and go high fiber. Vegetables, fruits, whole grains, and beans fit the bill perfectly.

HEALTHY EXAMPLES

By now, you already have a good idea of what this looks like on your plate, because the diet changes for weight loss are very much like those for controlling your blood sugar. Breakfast might start with veggie sausage or veggie bacon—that is, faux meats made of soy or wheat—followed by a big bowl of oatmeal or perhaps some fresh fruit. You would skip bacon, eggs, and ordinary bagels, which are stripped of fiber.

Lunch could be a sandwich made with sliced tomato, lettuce, and veggie deli slices on rye, or a pasta salad would be fine, too.

For dinner, you might try tomato or split pea soup followed by a vegetable stir-fry or shepherd's pie filled with chunky vegetables. In the process, you will avoid animal fat, have very little vegetable oil, and get all the fiber in those healthy vegetables.

For a between-meal snack, an apple or banana fits the bill nicely, while potato chips or nuts pack too much fat.

Vance

When Vance joined our study, he wanted to get his weight down to 210 to 225 pounds. Since he initially weighed in at 276 pounds, he had a ways to go. He stuck to the diet program, however, not worrying about calories or portions but paying close attention to the types of food he chose. Everything was vegan and low in fat. Also, in order to give the diet a good test, he agreed not to add any exercise for the first 6 months.

The pounds started to come off. Three months later, he weighed in at 251—a loss of 25 pounds in about 12 weeks. Friends couldn't help but notice, and many asked him what his secret was. After 6 months, he was down to 238. At the 14-month mark, he was at 217.

Nancy

Nancy began the study at 197 pounds. Like Vance, she changed her diet but kept her activity level the same to allow us to test what the diet change alone could do. Three months into the program, her weight was down by 14 pounds. After 6 months, she had lost 25 pounds, and

Not Exactly Health Food

A few years ago, I was running a study on diet and weight loss and found that a couple of our participants were chowing down on Twizzlers—the red candy that comes in long twists like licorice. When I asked why they were eating candy, they pointed out that the product is both vegan and low in fat. And sure enough, there's a friendly message printed on a package of Twizzlers Strawberry Twists:

> Did you know...
> Strawberry Twists are a low-fat candy! That's right, the same great-tasting Twizzlers you have known and loved are low in fat, as always. Nothing has changed.

A look at the ingredients list shows that, indeed, nothing *has* changed. Like other candies, it is basically a sugary concoction containing nothing that your body even remotely needs. Sugar is nowhere near as high in calories as fat, but it still provides more calories than you need.

at 14 months, she weighed 155 pounds—a loss of 42 pounds without counting calories.

FOODS THAT WORK MAGIC

These simple foods have surprising effects. Not only do they help you trim hundreds of calories off your daily menu, they also cause a fundamental change within the cells of your body. As you saw in Chapter 2, clinical tests have shown that they increase your body's after-meal calorie burn. The reason is this: As you change your diet, your insulin sensitivity begins to improve. That means that glucose has an easier time entering your cells to be burned for energy, rather than continuing to circulate in your blood.[3] The after-meal calorie burn is small, but it lasts for 3 or more hours after each meal, giving you an extra edge for losing weight.

APPETITE CONTROL

Barbara Rolls, PhD, a researcher at Pennsylvania State University, has proposed an innovative way of thinking about appetite control based on a concept called *energy density*.[4] Her studies have looked at what triggers satiety—the sense of fullness after meals—and shown how to plan meals to bring on a feeling of satiety earlier.

Surprisingly, what makes us stop eating does not seem to be the number of calories we have ingested, nor is it the amount of carbohydrate or protein in a meal. Rather, it is the *weight* of food we have taken in. It is as if your stomach has a scale, and once it registers a certain number of grams of food, it signals your brain that you have had enough.

We all tend to eat roughly the same weight of food each day. If your meals do not add up as they normally do, your appetite guides you to have a little more.

There's an effective weight-loss strategy in there. If the foods you eat contain a fair amount of water—soups or fruit, for example—they are heavy enough to tip your "stomach scale" and reduce your appetite.

Because the weight of these foods comes mainly from water, which has no calories, they tend to cut your total calorie intake for the day. These foods have a low energy density. That is, they have relatively few calories, even though they might have enough weight to convince your stomach that you've eaten quite a lot.

One important caveat: For some reason, simply drinking water will not turn off your appetite. Your stomach apparently reacts differently to heavy foods—which trigger an appetite shutoff—than to a drink of water, which does not.

Dr. Rolls proved this with an interesting lunchtime experiment. When research volunteers ate a casserole appetizer along with a glass of water, they ate about 400 calories at lunch. In a separate test, however, she stirred the glassful of water into the casserole to make soup. When she measured the participants' calorie intake afterward, she found it was cut to less than 300. The soup tricked their stomachs into shutting off their appetites.

Here are some tips for reducing the energy density of your meals.

- Soups are a great choice. They are filling but generally low in calories. Favor clear, low-sodium soups rather than creamy varieties.

- Add tomatoes, chickpeas, cucumbers, peppers, and other vegetables to turn a salad into a meal while keeping it low in calories. Use fat-free dressing, lemon juice, or apple cider vinegar rather than regular oily dressings.

- Apples, oranges, pears, mangoes, papayas, berries, and most other fruits are excellent choices for snacks, desserts, or a meal.

- Vegetables of virtually any variety are good choices. Adding chunky vegetables to salads and casseroles reduces their energy density in a very helpful way.

- Bean dishes are filling, but surprisingly modest in calories if they are made without added fat. Think of chili and casseroles.

- Go for whole grains. Rice beats rice cakes. Pasta beats bread. In each case, one is water-based and filling, while the other is airy and not filling at all. Old-fashioned oatmeal is a great breakfast choice.

Including these foods generously in your menu will accelerate your weight loss. There's an easy way to check the energy density of commercial food products: Just take a look at the label. If one serving has fewer calories than grams, it is a good choice. For example, the label on a can of black beans (below) shows that a serving has 90 calories and weighs 122 grams, so the beans are a good choice.

Black Beans

Nutrition Facts

Serving Size ½ cup (122 g)

Servings Per Container Approx 3½

Amount Per Serving: Calories 90, Calories from Fat 5

A can of spinach has 30 calories and 115 grams per serving, so it's also a winner. Each of these foods has less than 1 calorie per gram, so the weight of the food fills you up before the calories fill you out.

What about skinless chicken breast? One serving has 173 calories and weighs about 100 grams (3.5 ounces). Not a good choice. Aside from not being vegan or particularly low in fat (23 percent of calories), it has far more calories than grams.

A slice of bread may have 80 calories and weigh 32 grams. It has few calories but is very lightweight, so it is not filling. With more calories than grams, it is not especially helpful for weight loss.

I am not suggesting that you use energy density in place of the other diet guidelines in this book. Use it in addition to this program to ramp up the weight-loss power of your new menu. It will help you pick from among the allowed foods those that are the most filling with the fewest calories.

Again, the idea is simply to reduce the *energy density* of the foods you eat by choosing those that naturally contain a fair amount of water to fill you up and shut off your appetite.

STEER CLEAR OF LOW-CARB DIETS

Low-carbohydrate diets are popular, on and off. But they are potential disasters for anyone, especially for people with diabetes. They

Low-Carb Diets Can Worsen Cholesterol Levels

Weight loss lowers cholesterol levels. On average, each pound you lose lowers your cholesterol level about 1 point (that is, 1 mg/dl or 0.3 mmol/l),[5] so most weight-loss diets have a side benefit of improving your cholesterol test results. The exception is low-carbohydrate diets. They are so high in fat and cholesterol that they increase cholesterol levels for about one in every three dieters, some of whom have eventually experienced wildly high cholesterol levels and serious heart disease symptoms.[6, 7] There is no good reason to begin any low-carbohydrate, high-protein diet.

often bring short-term weight loss, but most of the weight quickly returns. Low-carb diets also have wildly unpredictable health effects. In research studies, as many as one-third of low-carb dieters have shown a significant increase in LDL ("bad") cholesterol. Some have had such high cholesterol levels that they have been forced to drop out of studies.

What's more, low-carb diets are usually high in protein. The animal protein that is commonly emphasized in these diets can be hard on your kidneys. Harvard researchers tracked kidney function in 1,624 women participating in the Nurses' Health Study, focusing especially on those who had any loss of kidney function at the start of the study. It turned out that the more animal protein the women consumed, the more kidney function they lost.[8] Given that about 40 percent of people with diabetes have already lost some kidney function, it makes good sense to protect yourself against further damage.[9] I strongly caution against any diets that recommend high-protein foods.

As you have seen, such diets are based on the outdated idea that avoiding carbohydrates is the key to glucose control. As you know by now, populations that make rice, noodles, and other carbohydrate-rich foods their diet staples actually have had very little obesity and very little diabetes.

Sometimes, when people blame "carbs" for their weight problems, they are thinking of cookies and cupcakes. But if you have ever looked at recipes for these products, you know that an enormous load of fat—

typically from butter or shortening—is usually lurking inside. So the carbohydrate in these products is really an innocent bystander; it's their load of fat that can fatten you up.

If you are stuck in the "carbs are fattening" mentality, let me share the results of an important study. National Institutes of Health researchers asked 19 overweight volunteers to follow a rigorously controlled low-carb diet and a low-fat diet at separate times—all the while under the watchful eyes of the NIH Metabolic Clinical Research Unit, where they lived throughout the experiment. Both diets had precisely the same number of calories; the difference was simply that one was low in fat and the other was low-carb. But the results were clear. The low-fat diet trimmed away roughly twice as much body fat, compared with the low-carb diet.[10]

Low-carb diets can cause weight loss over the short run, but there are far healthier ways to achieve that goal and to make weight loss last over the long run.

WHAT TO EXPECT

Everyone loses weight at his or her own pace. In our studies using low-fat vegan diets, weight loss averages about 1 pound per week. Adding exercise can increase your weight loss depending on your regimen.

You may find that you lose weight, then reach a plateau and stay there for a while. If that happens, see if there is something in your diet you can change, such as eliminating hidden sources of oil or boosting your fiber intake, or bringing in the low-energy-density foods we discussed above. Our bodies seem to have different plateaus depending on the fat content of our foods. That is to say, if you drop the fat content slightly, your weight will probably drop a bit, then plateau. If you drop the fat content more, you'll drop down to a new plateau.

The same thing works with fiber. Do a Quick Fiber Check (page 112), and if you're not up to 40 grams per day, try adding more beans, vegetables, fruits, and whole grains to your diet. You'll find that the combination of steering clear of fats and bringing in fiber helps trim away the pounds.

Take Your Time

If you have gradually gained weight over the years, let it come off gradually. Don't starve yourself in the hope of instant results. If you are on an optimal diet and are physically active, nature will take its course. As the weeks go by, you will not only be slimmer, you will also be healthier. Your cholesterol and blood pressure are likely to fall along with your blood glucose. As always, stay in close touch with your doctor so your medication doses can be revised as you regain your health.

CHAPTER 7

How to Test Yourself and Track Your Progress

In this chapter, we will look at the various tests that allow you to track your progress. The first one, glucose testing, is particularly important, but please read through the whole chapter. It will help you stay on the right path. We will start with blood tests and then look at other kinds of testing, including weight, blood pressure, and examinations of the eyes and feet.

GLUCOSE TESTING

Monitoring your blood sugar is important for controlling diabetes. Glucose is measured in milligrams per deciliter (mg/dl) in the United States and in millimoles per liter (mmol/l) in most of the rest of the world.

If you have type 1 diabetes or are using insulin for type 2 or gestational diabetes, you should check your glucose at least three times a day or according to whatever schedule your doctor recommends. If you have type 2 diabetes and are using oral medications, there is no optimal testing frequency. As a rule of thumb, however, when your diet, medications, exercise routine, or health status changes, it is important to test more frequently. If your doctor is not yet aware that you are about to make a change, now is the time to share that information. You should also discuss what to do if your blood glucose is too high or too low. As you begin a healthful diet, your numbers are likely to fall significantly.

Regular glucose testing is especially important if you are taking diabetes medications, particularly insulin or medications that cause your body to release insulin. The reason is that these are powerful drugs that actively push your blood sugar down. And you are now starting a powerful new diet. The combination of these treatments—drugs *and* diet (sometimes along with exercise)—may end up pushing your blood sugar too low.

I know what you may be thinking: Impossible! If all you have ever heard from your doctor is that your blood sugar is too high, it's hard to imagine it could fall too low. Well, it can. *The combination of a powerful diet and the diabetes medications you may already be on can be very strong.* In fact, your blood glucose can fall so low that you start to shake and sweat (see below for other symptoms). This is called hypoglycemia. In rare cases, people who make a major diet change or embrace a strenuous exercise program without backing off on medications find their blood sugar drops dangerously low—so low that they can lose consciousness. This is why it is essential that your doctor be made aware of the changes you are making—so your medication dosages can be altered if your blood glucose takes a nosedive.

Dangerous hypoglycemia is very unlikely if you are on no medications, and it is also unlikely if you are being treated with only metformin (Glucophage) or a thiazolidinedione, such as pioglitazone (Actos) or rosiglitazone (Avandia). However, hypoglycemia is *likely* to occur if you take any of the following drugs.

- Insulin (injected or pump)
- Glyburide (Micronase, Glynase, DiaBeta, or the combination drug Glucovance)
- Glipizide (Glucotrol)
- Glimepiride (Amaryl)
- Nateglinide (Starlix)
- Repaglinide (Prandin)

This is just a short list of medications that may put you at risk. Ask your doctor if the medications you are taking may cause hypoglycemia.

Although hypoglycemia is a sign that your body is regaining its insulin sensitivity—which is of course a good thing—it is also a sign that your medicines are now too strong and that you need to speak with your physician right away about adjusting your medication regimen. If your doctor has stopped your medications, hypoglycemia is very unlikely to occur.

Symptoms of hypoglycemia include:

- Shaking
- Sweating
- Hunger
- Anxiety
- Weakness
- Rapid heartbeat
- Dizziness or lightheadedness
- Sleepiness or confusion
- Difficulty speaking

If you experience these symptoms, check your blood sugar. If it is below 70 mg/dl (3.9 mmol/l) or whatever other benchmark value your doctor recommends, you need to eat something that raises your blood sugar quickly. If you notice symptoms while driving, pull over to a safe spot. And if you are unable to test your blood sugar or are unsure whether it is low, assume that it is low and have something to eat. Glucose tablets are a great choice. They are sold at all drugstores, and you will want to keep them in your purse or briefcase and in your glove compartment. If your blood sugar check shows you are hypoglycemic, you should take 15 grams of glucose. If you have typical glucose tablets with 4 grams of glucose each, you will need to take four tablets at once. Here are some other good choices.

- ½ cup (4 ounces) of any fruit juice
- ½ cup (4 ounces) of a regular (not diet) soft drink

- 5 or 6 pieces of hard candy

- 1 or 2 teaspoons of sugar

After 15 minutes, check your glucose again. If it is still below 70 mg/dl (3.9 mmol/l), have another serving, then check again in another 15 minutes. If you are within an hour of mealtime, go ahead and eat. If not, have a snack. Be sure to carry glucose tablets or a quick-energy food with you for emergencies, wear a medical identification bracelet, and be especially attentive to your glucose level during exercise, which can cause blood sugar to drop.

Hypoglycemia can also occur while you are asleep. Look for these signs.

- Nightmares or crying out

- Finding that your pajamas or sheets are damp from perspiration

- Awakening with unusual tiredness, confusion, or irritability

Carl's Hypoglycemic Episode

Carl had been taking metformin and glipizide for about 5 years, and his morning blood glucose values ranged between 120 and 150 mg/dl (6.7 and 8.3 mmol/l). He changed his diet with the hope of coming off his medications, and in fact, very soon after he began this program, his readings began to drop. After about 2 weeks, they were often under 100 mg/dl (5.6 mmol/l). Carl was delighted with such clear evidence that the changes were working.

About a month into the diet, he had an unusual experience. One morning at about 10:00 a.m., he found himself feeling unusually hungry. He always had a good appetite, but this was something different. He felt ravenous. Over the next several minutes, he started to tremble and broke into a sweat. "Oh, yes," he thought to himself. "This is what they told me might happen." He checked his blood glucose, and it was 65 mg/dl (3.6 mmol/l), which is lower than it should be. He had some orange juice and an early lunch. He telephoned his doctor, who reduced his glipizide dosage. Over the next several weeks, the episodes repeated several times. Eventually, his doctor stopped the glipizide altogether.

Carl's morning blood glucose readings stabilized at around 80 to 90 mg/dl (4.4 to 5.0 mmol/l). He never needed to go back on glipizide, and he never had another hypoglycemic episode.

If these occur, you can check for nighttime hypoglycemia. Simply set your alarm for about 2:00 or 3:00 a.m. and check your blood sugar a few nights in a row. Consult your doctor to see if you need a medication change.

Hypoglycemia does not mean there is anything wrong with your diet. Rather, it means that the medication regimen you are on has become too strong for you. The next step is to contact your physician or other caregiver, who will probably reduce your medication dosages or eliminate one or more drugs. Get in touch with your doctor as soon as possible—the same day the episode occurs. Do not put it off, because the hypoglycemic episodes are likely to recur until your medications are reduced.

To track your blood sugar, use a logbook or a simple grid like the one below.

Blood Glucose						
DATE	MEDICATION REGIMEN	EARLY	BREAKFAST	LUNCH	DINNER	LATE
			/	/	/	
			/	/	/	
			/	/	/	
			/	/	/	
			/	/	/	
			/	/	/	
			/	/	/	
			/	/	/	
			/	/	/	
			/	/	/	
			/	/	/	
			/	/	/	
			/	/	/	
			/	/	/	
			/	/	/	
			/	/	/	
			/	/	/	

Note: It is especially helpful to check your blood glucose before meals. Mark these numbers to the left of the slash marks. Mark after-meal values to the right of the slash marks.

MAKING SENSE OF GLUCOSE

Blood glucose values are a bit like the stock market: Although they generally follow a trend, they can bounce around from day to day. Certain situations can trigger an unexpected rise. Any sort of illness or infection can boost your blood glucose; even a minor upper respiratory illness or a scraped foot can cause a significant jump in your numbers. Stress can, too, due to the action of stress-related hormones.

Having some up-and-down swings in blood sugar is normal, but if your glucose remains high day after day, your risk of complications is higher than it would be if your glucose level were better controlled. The American Diabetes Association recommends that people with diabetes use the following guidelines for blood glucose levels.

• Fasting or before meals: 80 to 130 mg/dl (4.4 to 7.2 mmol/l)

• One to 2 hours after a meal: below 180 mg/dl (10.0 mmol/l)

THE DAWN PHENOMENON
AND THE SOMOGYI EFFECT

You may occasionally be surprised to find that your blood glucose is higher in the morning than it was when you went to bed the night before. Or perhaps you checked your glucose in the early morning and then went back to sleep, only to find that it had risen while you slept. How is this possible?

No, sugarplums dancing in your head had nothing to do with it. The fact is, your body constantly monitors the amount of glucose in your bloodstream and adjusts it from time to time. Glucose is vital to your body's functioning—especially to the workings of your brain—so your body has a way of increasing your blood glucose when it gets a bit low. In the early-morning hours—typically between 5:00 and 9:00 a.m.— hormones (growth hormone, cortisol, and catecholamines) cause your liver to release glucose into the bloodstream. These hormones can also interfere with insulin's efforts to remove glucose from the blood. This "dawn phenomenon" can noticeably raise your blood sugar.[1]

A similar reaction can occur when a person using long-acting insulin has an unusual blood glucose dip in the middle of the night. Let's say, for example, that you miss your usual late-night snack, and the insulin you are taking forces your glucose level too low. Once again, your natural hormones will compensate, raising your blood sugar. This is called the Somogyi effect. It is different from the dawn phenomenon in that it is triggered by an overly low blood sugar level occurring in the middle of the night.

Although your body has a system for controlling your blood sugar, it is a bit imprecise. Your blood sugar can still run too low or too high despite your body's best efforts, and you will occasionally see a high or low level that you cannot explain.

HEMOGLOBIN A1C

As discussed in Chapter 1, the main test for assessing your progress is hemoglobin A1C. Your A1C level should be checked every 6 months, or every 3 months if your diet, medications, or general health is changing or if previous values have been too high. If your A1C is high, your doctor will be concerned, and you should be, too. If it is low, you are doing well. To give you a frame of reference, the American Diabetes Association says that most people with diabetes should keep their A1C below 7 percent. A lower target, say 6.5 percent, makes sense if you can get there without risking hypoglycemia (that is, if you are not on medications that are likely to cause hypoglycemia). If you do tend to have frequent hypoglycemic episodes, your caregiver may recommend a less stringent target, say 8.0 percent, in order to keep your blood glucose from falling too low.

A typical oral diabetes medication brings A1C down by an average of about 1 point or a bit less. The effect of a good diet on A1C varies depending on how good your control is when you start, how well you follow the diet, and how much excess weight you lose. Your result will also be affected by exercise, genetics, and other factors.

The biggest drops we have seen in short-term research studies are around 4 points in approximately 6 months. These are seen in people whose A1Cs were high (say, 9 or 10) to begin with. People whose A1Cs are in the 7 to 8 range are likely to have a drop averaging between 1 and 2 points. People who continue to lose weight beyond this time could have an even greater drop, assuming they were not already in the normal range.

The higher your A1C, the greater your risk of circulatory problems. Evidence suggests that keeping A1C low is particularly important for the health of your eyes and kidneys and for preventing nerve symptoms.

From your heart's standpoint, a 1-point increase on the A1C scale—from 7 to 8 or 8 to 9, for example—brings about a 20 percent increase in your risk of heart problems over about a decade.[2] In other words, if you had a 10 percent risk of having a heart attack sometime in the next decade, a 1-point rise in your A1C, maintained over the whole decade, would boost your risk to 12 percent. A 2-point rise would mean a 14 percent risk, and so on. What these numbers tell us is that A1C is important and that by all means, you will want to aim to get your A1C down. However, A1C is not the sole key to good health. To stop diabetes from attacking your heart and blood vessels, you will also want to focus on your blood pressure, cholesterol, and weight. Needless to say, your doctor can and should track these values with you.

CHOLESTEROL

Your doctor will check your cholesterol at regular intervals, at least once a year. As you will see in Chapter 12, high levels of cholesterol in the blood can damage your heart, major blood vessels, and the delicate blood vessels of the eyes and kidneys. Here are the numbers to aim for.[3]

Total cholesterol. According to most authorities, total cholesterol should be below 200 mg/dl (5.2 mmol/l). I suggest you aim for a considerably lower goal, however. First of all, the average cholesterol level in the United States is hovering around 200 mg/dl, and in a country where heart attacks are the cause of death for half the population, you do not want to be anywhere near average! In large population studies, it is clear that the lower your cholesterol, the lower your risk of heart problems, until you reach a threshold of about 150 mg/dl (3.9 mmol/l).

My suggestion is to use that as your goal rather than the more permissive "official" figure.

Low-density lipoprotein (LDL) cholesterol. LDL cholesterol is often called bad cholesterol because it raises your risk of heart problems and other blood vessel complications. According to most authorities, your LDL should be below 100 mg/dl (2.6 mmol/l). Your risk of heart problems drops as LDL decreases, until you reach a level of approximately 40 mg/dl (1.0 mmol/l).[4]

High-density lipoprotein (HDL) cholesterol. HDL cholesterol is often called good cholesterol because it carries cholesterol out of the body. Some evidence suggests that the higher your HDL cholesterol, the better. Current goals are to have an HDL level above 40 mg/dl (1.0 mmol/l) for men and above 50 mg/dl (1.34 mmol/l) for women.

Some doctors, however, interpret HDL in the context of your total cholesterol concentration: In this case, a favorable HDL reading would be at least one-third of your total cholesterol. For example, if your total cholesterol is 150, a healthy HDL would be 50 or above. This is an important consideration because many people who follow healthful diets do not have much of *any* kind of cholesterol—LDL, HDL, or anything else.

Recent evidence has called the importance of HDL into question. Although lowering LDL cholesterol does reduce your risk of heart problems, raising HDL does not seem to make any difference.

Triglycerides. Triglycerides are tiny fat particles transported in the bloodstream. Normal triglyceride concentration is less than 150 mg/dl (1.7 mmol/l).

See Chapter 12 for information on controlling cholesterol and triglycerides.

TRACKING YOUR BLOOD PRESSURE

Maintaining healthy blood pressure is extremely important. As you can imagine, increased pressure inside your arteries can damage the arteries themselves, as well as your heart, eyes, kidneys, and nerves. The longer your blood pressure stays high, the more damage it can do.

Problems can travel in the other direction, too: Damage to the kidneys can lead to high blood pressure. The reason is that your kidneys play an important role in regulating your blood pressure, and if they have been assaulted by diabetes, they can lose some of their ability to do this.

In Chapter 12, we will look at how diet affects blood pressure. For now, here are your targets.

Normal blood pressure is less than 120/80 millimeters of mercury (mmHg). If you have high blood pressure, your caregiver will work with you to reduce it to below 140/90, and to below 130/80 if you can get there without serious medication side effects. If you are pregnant, the target will be 120–160/80–105, aiming to protect both you and your baby.[5]

It goes without saying that diet changes are key for controlling blood pressure and can often make medications unnecessary. The same plant-based diet that helps you lose weight and brings down your blood sugar will also help you control your blood pressure.

Have your blood pressure checked regularly. If it is not where it should be, take another look at your diet and speak with your doctor about what, if any, additional treatments you may need. A healthful diet and the weight loss it brings can also mean that your caregiver will cut back on blood pressure medicines you may be on, or stop them altogether. But don't stop your medicines on your own.

CHECKING YOUR KIDNEY HEALTH

Because your kidneys can easily be affected by diabetes, your doctor will check your kidney health with a simple urine test at least once a year. The goal is to see whether your kidneys are losing protein, specifically a protein molecule called albumin. Albumin itself is not especially important. What is important is that if it shows up in your urine, it is a sign that your kidneys have been affected by diabetes and are not holding on to albumin as they should. Albumin losses of greater than 30 milligrams over 24 hours are considered abnormal. Your doctor will also check your blood for creatinine and estimate your glomerular filtration rate and will interpret the results of these tests for you. For more on factors that influence kidney health, see Chapter 13.

OTHER ROUTINE LABORATORY TESTS

Your doctor will run other tests to track your progress. The following are two very common ones.

Complete blood count (CBC). This test shows the state of your blood cells. Many people with diabetes develop anemia, meaning they have fewer red blood cells than they should. A complete blood count lets your doctor easily check this and many other measures. If your blood count is low, your doctor will investigate the reasons for it, which could include kidney disease, iron deficiency, use of certain medications, abnormal bleeding, or other factors.

Chemistry panel. A routine chemistry panel is also known by several other names. It assesses your overall health, with a special focus on the status of your kidneys and liver and lets doctors check for potential adverse effects from medications.

There is no reason to despair if any of your laboratory values are not where they should be, but it is definitely a reason to take action. You will want to optimize your diet and work with your doctor to plot a course for tracking the effectiveness of your overall health regimen.

TAKING STOCK OF YOUR DIET

I would like to shift gears now and look at your diet and overall health. First, let's take a minute to make sure that your diet is going according to plan.

- Are your foods vegan? You know you are doing well if there are no foods of animal origin on your plate, not even little bits of fish, fat-free milk, or egg white—nothing. If you have done this right, there is *no* animal fat, *no* cholesterol, and *no* animal protein in your diet. Your menu is built from plant foods, and it is rich in fiber and all the healthy nutrients the plant kingdom brings you. If you need a refresher on why you are doing this, please take another look at Chapter 4.

- Are your meals all low in fat? It is important to really keep fats and oils to an absolute minimum. Be careful with nuts and nut products.

- Are your foods low GI? The main problem foods are sugar, corn syrup (a common sweetener in processed foods), white and whole wheat breads (favor rye and pumpernickel), and baking potatoes (choose sweet potatoes and yams).

QUICK FIBER CHECK

One way to help gauge how you are doing is with the Quick Fiber Check. It is a handy little tool, and I suggest that you do one about once a week as you begin this new approach to eating. Scoring is simple and takes only a minute or two to learn. Soon, estimating the fiber content of virtually everything in the supermarket will be a snap. You will also see if you are getting enough fiber in your daily menu. It does not take long, and it will help you see if you are on track.

First, take a minute to jot down everything you ate or drank for 1 full day on the form below. I will explain below how to fill in the fiber column.

Food (one food or ingredient per line)   **Fiber**

_____   _____

_____   _____

_____   _____

_____   _____

_____   _____

_____   _____

_____   _____

_____   _____

_____   _____

_____   _____

_____   _____

_____   _____

_____   _____

                                                        Total _____

Then, next to each food, note its fiber score, using the following guide.

Beans: For each serving of beans or lentils (one serving = ½ cup) or any food that includes about this amount of beans or lentils as an ingredient, give yourself a 7. One cup of soy milk or ½ cup of tofu (both made from soybeans) rates a 3.

Vegetables: For each serving of vegetables (one serving = 1 cup), give yourself a 4. An exception is lettuce, for which 1 cup scores a 2. A potato with skin scores a 4; without the skin, a 2.

Fruit: For each medium piece of fruit (e.g., an apple, orange, or banana; 1 cup applesauce; a banana smoothie), mark a 3. For 1 cup of juice, mark a 1.

Grains: For each piece of white bread, bagel, or equivalent, score a 1. Whole grain breads score a 2, as does 1 cup of cooked pasta. One cup of rice scores a 1 for white and a 3 for brown. One cup of cooked oatmeal scores a 4. Score a 3 for typical ready-to-eat cereals, a 1 for highly processed and colored cereals, and an 8 for bran.

Soda, water: Score a 0.

Interpreting Your Score

Total your fiber score and let's see how you are doing.

Less than 20: You need more fiber in your diet. As it is, your appetite will be hard to control, and you may have occasional constipation. Boosting fiber will help tame your appetite and cut your risk of many health problems.

20–39: You are doing better than most people in Western countries, but as you bring more fiber into your diet, you will find that it makes foods more satisfying and cuts your calorie intake a bit.

40 or more: Congratulations! You have plenty of healthy fiber in your diet to control your appetite and help keep you healthy. Fiber also reduces your risk of developing cancer, heart disease, diabetes, and digestive problems.

CHECKING YOUR WEIGHT

Of all the things that predict success in dealing with diabetes, leaving behind excess weight is among the most important. The strategy outlined in Chapter 6 is a highly effective way to go about it.

Here are some tips for tracking your progress.

- First, track your weight. Some people who have been overweight for a long time have not gone near a scale in years. If that sounds like you, give it another try. It is essential to know if you are losing. If you are not losing weight, it is time to change course. Usually, that means tuning up your diet. Weight loss is sometimes difficult, and genetic tendencies do play a role, but your diet is one thing you really can control.

- Use the same scale each time you weigh yourself. Different scales can give dramatically different readings.

- Check your weight at the same time of day each time. With food and water intake, you can easily gain and lose a few pounds in the course of a day. Usually, you will be heavier in the evening.

- In gauging the success of your weight loss, about 1 pound per week is a healthful goal. It is about what you can expect if you follow the diet presented in this book without doing particularly vigorous exercise. Slower weight loss is also fine as long as you are moving in the right direction.

- Do not rely on exercise alone for weight loss. A healthful diet change can easily trim 300 to 400 calories a day off your daily menu, but burning that many calories through exercise means walking or running *3 or 4 miles a day*. Exercise is important, but it cannot begin to take the place of diet changes.

CHECKING YOUR EYES

At least once a year, you should have an eye examination by an ophthalmologist to check for any sign of retinopathy. These changes cannot be detected by an ordinary eye examination with a doctor's ophthalmoscope or during an optometric examination for eyeglasses. Also be sure to see an eye specialist if you have had any changes in your vision.

If you smoke, tell your eye doctor. Yes, you will get a lecture, and it is time to listen up if you are still smoking. See Chapter 13 for information on the effects of nutrition on eye health.

CHECKING YOUR FEET

Foot problems are common in diabetes. If your blood glucose has been poorly controlled, you are at risk of developing neuropathy—nerve damage—which means you may not be aware of small injuries to your feet. Wound healing may be slowed as well. Small injuries can gradually worsen and become infected.

For this reason, you not only want to get your diet into shape by following the guidelines in this book, you also want to have your doctor check your feet at least once a year. The examination will include a check for sensation using a thin plastic thread, a check of your vibratory sense with a tuning fork, and a thorough check for any signs of damage to your skin. Take the advice of Mary Ellen Wolfe, RN, a nurse working with George Washington University, who recommends that you take off your shoes and socks at every doctor's visit to be sure your doctor does not forget to examine your feet.

STAYING HEALTHY

No matter how healthy you get, you should still keep an eye on your glucose, A1C, and cholesterol; blood pressure; weight; eyes; and feet. But I hope as you tune up your diet and lifestyle, that it's all you will be doing—just confirming that all is just as it should be.

CHAPTER 8

A Perfect Diet in an Imperfect World

It is not always easy to follow a perfect diet in an imperfect world. There will be times when those you depend on—restaurants, airlines, co-workers, and even family members—have little understanding of or interest in healthy foods. This chapter is dedicated to these situations. I will cover dining out, travel, social situations, working with your doctor, and dealing with family members. When life throws you a curveball, I will show you how to step up to the plate and stay in the game.

DINING OUT

Dining out is part of life, and you ought to be able to enjoy a night on the town with friends or loved ones without missing a beat on your new healthy diet. Luckily, many restaurant menus offer plenty of healthy selections. Unfortunately, others are limited. Often the key to success lies in where you go and what you order when you get there. Here are a few tips.

First, think international. In Mediterranean countries, Asia, Africa, and Latin America, the traditional dietary staples are grains, vegetables, legumes, and fruits. Not surprisingly, all of these regions have historically had much lower rates of diabetes than North America and Western Europe. When you choose from the best of what these cuisines have to offer, dinner out can be both healthy and delicious.

Italian restaurants are everywhere, and they would love to serve you spaghetti with a marinara or arrabbiata sauce, minestrone, pasta e fagiole (a traditional soup made with pasta and beans), healthy salads, chunky vegetable-and-tomato pizza, grilled asparagus, and steamed spinach. Because their foods are usually made to order, it is a snap for chefs to minimize oil, leave off cheese, serve sauces on the side, and so on.

Mexican restaurants are ubiquitous in North America and serve bean or vegetable burritos, veggie fajitas, rice, and salads. Most have stopped using lard to make their beans, and all are happy to skip the cheese. Top foods with salsa if you like.

Latin American cuisine comes in other wonderful varieties, too. Cuban and Brazilian restaurants offer black bean dishes, rice, plantains, salads, salsa, and other healthful fare.

Chinese restaurants will get you started with vegetable spring rolls or vegetable pot stickers and various healthy soups. Favor the steamed, not fried, items. Skip the meat dishes and get right to the long list of savory vegetable main dishes made with tofu (also known as bean curd), green beans, broccoli, spinach, and other healthful ingredients. The danger in Chinese restaurants, as in most eating establishments, is overexuberance with the use of oil. Ask that your food be prepared with as little oil as possible and have your main dish along with plenty of rice, preferably brown rice.

Japanese restaurants are among the very best choices when it comes to healthful dining. Sushi chefs are delighted to transform carrots, cucumbers, radishes, sweet potatoes, and other simple ingredients into edible delights. Have them along with miso soup, salads, seaweed, and various appetizers.

Thai and **Vietnamese** restaurants serve many meatless dishes that include rice, soft noodles, vegetables, and tofu along with wonderful sauces.

Indian restaurants are mixed. While vegetarian diets are traditional and highly respected among many Indians, the use of oil and dairy products often puts them in the no-go zone. Your best choices are soups, rice dishes, and vegetable curries prepared with minimal oil.

Ethiopian restaurants are common in major cities. Because some religious groups in Ethiopia follow vegan diets during certain days of the week and certain times of the year, the restaurants serve many dishes made with chickpeas, split peas, lentils, green beans, peppers, and delightful spices. They will be happy to serve you all their vegan items on a large platter for a wonderful dinner.

American restaurants, family restaurants, and even steakhouses have salad bars and offer vegetable plates. Many serve pasta dishes even when they are not on the menu.

Second, ask for what you want. If what you are looking for is not on the menu, do not be afraid to ask. Most restaurateurs will gladly alter their main offerings to accommodate a special request. If you would like cheese and bacon bits left off your salad, if you would like a vegetable plate, or if you would like your pasta topped with tomato sauce instead of meat sauce, by all means, ask. You will not only get a better meal, you will also help the restaurant management understand how to better serve patrons like you.

As I noted above, restaurant kitchens often overdo it with oils, so ask your server how foods are prepared and request that your meal be made with as little oil as possible. In Italian restaurants, spinach and broccoli are often sautéed, but they can also be steamed. The same goes for most Asian vegetable dishes.

Sauces and condiments can always be served on the side. This goes for pasta sauces, salad dressings, brown sauces used in Asian cuisine, spreads used on sandwiches, and similar items.

Ask for what you want. You will be glad you did.

A Breakfast Trick

Most restaurants will gladly serve a healthful bowl of oatmeal for breakfast and will top it with strawberries, blueberries, or cinnamon. But once in a while, you'll find precious little at eateries that are busy serving bacon and eggs. Here's a trick:

Ask the server to have the cook throw some tomatoes, spinach, and mushrooms on the grill. Maybe some asparagus, too. Chefs are accustomed to stuffing them into omelets; now, you're just having them without the eggs! With a side of rye toast (no butter, of course), you're set.

Fast Food

Fast food is rarely a top choice when the priority is healthy eating. On the other hand, these chains are big businesses that understand the growing demand for healthy food choices. More and more often, you find offerings on their menus that fit into a healthy diet.

Taco Bell's bean burrito—if you hold the cheese—is entirely vegan. If you like, add tomatoes, lettuce, or jalapeño chile peppers.

Burger King offers a veggie burger that is much lower in fat than its other sandwiches and will also gladly sell you a Veggie Whopper with all the toppings but without the burger. Submarine sandwich shops will gladly leave off the meat and cheese and pile on the lettuce, tomato, cucumbers, spinach, and peppers, plus a dash of red wine vinegar. And they will even toast it for you. Denny's offers a veggie burger, and most family restaurants serve plenty of side vegetables that together make a good vegetable plate.

Some fast-food restaurants offer salad bars. With chickpeas, three-bean salad, cherry tomatoes, and chopped vegetables, a salad becomes a hearty meal.

In that vein, one of the best ways to get healthy food fast is to stop at any large supermarket and patronize its salad bar. A wealth of great choices is right at your fingertips.

NANCY'S AND VANCE'S EXPERIENCES

Nancy often dined with friends who liked good food and good restaurants. I encouraged her to choose ethnic cuisine—Chinese, Japanese, Italian, or Thai, for example. Unfortunately, that was not what most of her friends had in mind, and they felt uncomfortable knowing she would not eat unhealthy things.

When she headed out to join friends at a restaurant that might not be very accommodating, she often had a snack in advance so she would not be starving when she got there. When she went to open houses during the winter holidays, she often volunteered to bring a fruit and vegetable tray.

On a vacation to Iceland, she packed granola bars and individual soy milk packages in her luggage, to supplement the local food, and got by just fine.

"I am tempted sometimes, especially when I am stressed or over-tired. I talk myself out of it," she said.

She found it helpful to keep things in perspective. "You have to decide what your priorities are," she explained. "I didn't want to suffer from the effects of the disease. I wanted to stop the progression. I didn't even think about reversing it. And now I'm a walking advertisement for the program. People keep asking me how I've done it. I've described it in detail to probably 40 people."

When Vance dined out, he looked for veggie burgers, fresh steamed vegetables, and pasta without cheese and oils. His challenge was sports stadiums. "I love going to baseball and football games, where french fries, hot dogs, and soft drinks are about all that's offered. It would be great to be able to bring in healthy food or even just some carrot sticks and a bottle of water, but usually they don't allow any food to be brought in. So at first I stuck to pretzels, popcorn, and Crystal Light. At a game in Seattle, I smelled the fish and fries, and it was hard to resist," he said.

Veggie hot dogs and burgers came to Vance's rescue. Although they are not necessarily the ultimate dining experience, they are a major improvement on the foods they replace, and more and more stadiums, movie theaters, and other venues are starting to sell them.

TRAVEL

Travel presents challenges no matter what kind of diet you follow. Here are a few ways to help keep your new eating plan on track.

Choose restaurants wisely. As you have seen, there are usually plenty of vegan choices at nonvegan restaurants, particularly those that feature international cuisine. Even some fast-food places can rise to the occasion.

You might go online to check out vegan and vegetarian restaurants in cities you are planning to visit. A Web site called Happy Cow's Veg-etarian Guide (happycow.net) lists them by location, but call before you go; restaurants are forever starting up and shutting down. There's no reason to limit yourself to these restaurants, though; almost any eating establishment should be able to accommodate you.

Plan before you fly. When you are booking an international flight (or generally up to 48 hours before your flight), request a vegan meal. You will get a healthy meal and will often be served first.

On domestic flights, most meal service has gone by the wayside, so you might pick up some easy-to-pack snacks at a health food store or supermarket. Vegan deli slices are great sandwich fillers and resist spoiling. A pack of hummus with pita bread, a few pieces of fresh fruit, some baby carrots, instant soup cups (flight attendants will gladly provide hot water), or a small pop-top can of chickpeas can be lifesavers.

SOCIAL EVENTS

It can be tough to stick to the plan at parties, even when you know you will regret a slip in the morning. If you arrive at a party unprepared, there may well be nothing available that you can eat. With a bit of planning, though, you can celebrate without leaving the healthy path you are on. Here are some ideas.

Offer to bring a healthy dish. Let's say you have been asked to the home of some friends for dinner, and you have no idea what they will serve. Here is what I suggest: When you get the invitation or as soon thereafter as possible, call your hosts to let them know that you have changed your diet and that you do not want to put them to any trouble. Say that you would like to bring something, such as a low-fat hummus dip or an exotic fruit salad. I can almost guarantee that your hosts will say there is no need to worry and you need not bring anything because there will be plenty to eat. Now, regardless of what they were really thinking, you have alerted them to your needs without imposing in the slightest.

If you are reluctant to let your hosts know, do not be. They will be much more embarrassed if they find out after the fact that they served a dinner with nothing you wanted to eat. Besides, you are very likely to find that other guests—and even your hosts—are making similar diet changes.

Bring a healthy gift. Instead of the usual bottle of wine, why not arrive with a healthful food gift? A fruit basket, a loaf of artisan pumpernickel bread, or a healthy party dip (you can find all of these at health food stores) will delight your hosts and ensure that you have something to eat.

Avoid arriving hungry. If you arrive ravenous, you will be drawn to the platters of unhealthful foods. If you eat something before you arrive, you will be fine.

Carry a plate. Party guests with nothing in their hands are inviting others to offer them something. Make yourself a plate with a few crudités or a bit of bread, and no one will be inclined to offer you foods you do not want to eat.

AT THE DOCTOR'S OFFICE

Medical care is a partnership; you and your doctor need to work together to best meet your needs. This is true at any time, but especially when you are in the process of changing your diet. The fact is, your diabetes will probably be improving, and you will need to ratchet down your medications.

Some doctors are not easy to reach, and even if you have your doctor's attention, that does not mean he or she wants to engage in a conversation about nutrition. Some physicians show little interest in the topic, while others have frankly outdated or untested ideas about it.

I suggest you lend a copy of this book to your physician with a sticky note flagging Chapter 14. It was written for doctors and shows them how they can best help you.

You can help by holding up your end of the partnership. That means following your doctor's advice (provided it is sound and you agree with it), letting him or her know how you are doing, calling promptly if your blood glucose drops below 70 mg/dl (3.9 mmol/l) or whatever other criterion is set, and taking a vitamin B_{12} supplement so he or she will not worry about your developing any sort of deficiency. The truth is, your nutrition is much better on a vegan diet than on an omnivorous diet, but a knowledgeable doctor will want to be sure you are getting your B_{12}. A supplement will easily take care of that.

In the vast majority of cases, doctors are delighted when their patients improve their diets. They are all the more delighted when they see the improvements on the scale and in laboratory results.

One of our research volunteers thought his doctor would be skeptical about his plans. They talked about little aside from blood tests and prescriptions during his appointments. To his surprise, however, when the doctor found out he was starting a vegan diet, she was delighted. "That will probably help you a great deal," she said. And indeed, it did. Within 6 months, he lost 30 pounds, was able to stop one of his two diabetes medications, and was continuing to improve week by week. His doctor had no formal education in nutrition, but she knew success when she saw it. She now recommends the same diet to other diabetes patients.

LOVED ONES WHO HELP AND HURT

Sometimes our friends and family members help us stay on a healthy path. When we are not enthusiastic about exercising, they encourage us by going with us. When we are tempted by some less-than-healthful food, they shore up our resolve.

Improving our diets is like quitting smoking or breaking any other habit: We need our family's support. But sometimes, intentionally or unintentionally, our loved ones are not so helpful. They may not be aware of the risks of a bad diet, or perhaps they are all too aware and are struggling with unhealthful habits of their own. They may even try to sabotage your efforts to break bad habits.

If the problem is that your loved ones simply do not have much information about healthful diets, lend them this book. If they are not eager readers, try this little trick: Put a sticky note or bookmark at any page you think they would find of special interest. They will be drawn to that section, and once they start reading, they will probably continue.

If family members tease you about your eating habits, remind them how important your health is to you. Explain that it is tough for you to have unhealthful foods around and that you really need their help.

Ideally, they will join you in your new, healthy way of eating. If they just will not change, then at a minimum, they must keep their food separate and not tease or tempt you with unhealthy items.

GOOD FOOD FOR THE WHOLE FAMILY

If you are preparing meals for your family and they are balking at new foods, do not despair. It is natural to be cautious about anything new. Present healthful foods without pushing them and recognize that it often takes a couple of tries before a new item really catches on.

I suggest that you not fix healthy meals for yourself and less-than-healthy meals for your spouse or children. Some people do this, figuring they cannot change others' bad habits. But remember this: Not only will introducing healthful foods to your family bring you some very important allies, it will benefit your loved ones as well as you.

The very best situation is when the whole family decides to change together. There is no health reason for anyone to eat animal-derived foods, fatty foods, or sugary foods. Yes, these foods are everywhere in modern societies, but they are the principal reason for the epidemics of overweight, heart disease, cancer, and other health problems in North America and much of the rest of the world. When the whole family makes the same diet change, they all get the same advantage.

One good way to break through resistance is to ask your family members to try a short-term diet change with you as an experiment. Say that you'd like to try new and healthy ways of eating for just 3 weeks, and you would like them to join you. Most people will try anything for a short period. By the time 3 weeks have passed, they will have sorted out the new foods they like and will be ready for more.

When introducing healthful foods to children, it is generally best to stick to simple, familiar items. Some children may not yet care for exotic vegetables, but they will easily gravitate to fruit of all kinds, as well as corn, green beans, carrots, peas, and other simple foods. Avoid wrangling with a child who is reluctant to try a new food. Sometimes altering the form of the food makes a huge difference. A child who does not care for the texture of cooked spinach may like fresh spinach

as part of a salad. Steamed broccoli and cauliflower may be intimidat-
ing, but they may be perfectly acceptable when chopped and added to
a soup or stew. Kids may not go for lentil loaf, but they love veggie
burgers and hot dogs and sandwiches made with vegetarian deli slices.

It always helps to present choices. Would your children prefer baked
beans or lentil soup? Would they prefer their veggie burgers cut into
halves or quarters? The idea is to give kids a sense of control while all
the possibilities are good ones.

In some families, food is a symbol of affection. Parents stuff their
children with cookies and gooey desserts, as if love could be measured
in calories. Whatever the motivation, none of this does you one bit of
good. Find other ways to express affection. A book, a walk, a trip to
the movies—there is no shortage of meaningful gifts.

HEALTHFUL FOODS IN AN UNHEALTHY WORLD

A visitor from another planet might well conclude that modern civiliza-
tion has no perceptible interest in healthful diets. Fast-food restaurants—
and regular restaurants—carry lots of fatty, cholesterol-laden meals and
far fewer healthful choices. Television commercials push endless less-
than-healthful snacks. Convenience stores and snack machines offer
lots of what you do not want and precious little of what you do want.
Sometimes, you may feel like a person who is trying to quit smoking
but is trapped in a bar where cigarettes are free.

In large part, you would be right, but truly, there are also plenty of
healthful options. For every convenience store selling unhealthy food,
there is a supermarket with an ever-expanding range of great food products. For every restaurant that refuses to serve anything health-conscious
eaters would look for, there are a dozen that offer good choices. The
range of health-oriented cookbooks is truly enormous, and it is now
easier than ever to follow a healthful diet. Friends and family members—
even those who do not follow healthy diets themselves—all know that
what you are doing is worth supporting.

CHAPTER 9

Troubleshooting

How are you doing with your new way of eating? Are you reaching your weight-loss goals? Are your glucose and A1C coming down? Is your cholesterol improving?

If you are having any sort of trouble, this chapter will guide you through the most common problem spots.

NOT LOSING WEIGHT

People who begin low-fat, vegan diets typically lose weight easily. In our research studies, the average rate is about 1 pound per week. Some people lose more quickly, others a bit more slowly, but a pound a week is a good pace. If you think about what this means over a year's time, the result is impressive, particularly since you are free of the yo-yo syndrome that comes with diets based on calorie restrictions. Because this is not a short-term, starve-yourself-thin diet, it does not cause hunger, so there is no rebound bingeing. Gradual, healthy weight loss is what you can expect. Sometimes losing weight can be a bit like following the stock market. There are fluctuations up and down, but the trend should be clear. If you are not losing weight, it is time to take action. Here are the steps to take.

Get back to the basics. Be sure you are following the guidelines in Chapter 4 and giving it 100 percent. That means no animal products in your diet at all. If your diet includes fish or cheese, for example, your weight-loss efforts will be hampered.

Check for hidden oils. Packaged foods should include no more than 3 grams of fat per serving. If you frequently eat at restaurants, try to assess to what extent they are packing oils into their meals. If you are unsure (or your server is unsure), ask for foods to be steamed rather than fried or sautéed and that any sauces or dressings be served on the side. See Chapter 8.

Do a Quick Fiber Check. If you check your fiber intake (see page

Don't Get Sidetracked by Rationalizations

Sometimes people who are not losing weight blame genetics, lack of exercise, or something else for their problem. Genetics and exercise do play roles, of course. But if you are not losing weight, the problem is nearly always dietary.

Once, en route from Washington to London, I was busily typing away on my laptop, writing an article about diet changes for weight loss. The passenger next to me happened to see what I was typing and took an interest in the topic. He had been overweight for several years and wanted to see what I might suggest. I explained our research findings about how diet changes could cause lasting weight loss. I pointed out that the key seemed to be changing the types of foods we eat. I launched into a discussion of the benefits of vegetables, fruits, beans, and whole grains and the wonderful meals they can become.

"That's interesting," he said, "but I think I just need to exercise more. That's my real problem. I used to exercise a lot, but lately, I've been so busy." He brushed aside the whole topic of food.

A few minutes later, the flight attendant came by with the meal service. She served him a ham-and-cheese sandwich, a bag of chips, and a soft drink, which he shoveled into his mouth without a word. I suspect he did not realize that it would take a very long session at the gym to burn away those unnecessary calories. The airline also served vegetarian meals, which would have been a much better choice.

Shortly thereafter, I was talking to a patient with Stanley Talpers, MD, an internist on the faculty of the George Washington University School of Medicine in Washington, D.C. The patient said he hadn't been losing weight, and he figured that he just needed to walk more. Dr. Talpers encouraged him to get his diet in order first because, he said, "to lose a pound by walking, you'd have to walk to Baltimore." It is true. Exercise is beneficial, and I strongly recommend it. But a lack of exercise is not the primary reason for weight problems, and exercise can never take the place of a healthful diet.

112) and find that you are eating less than 40 grams of fiber per day, you'll want to bring in more beans, vegetables, and fruits.

If your diet is vegan, low in fat, and high in fiber, it is very hard not to lose weight. Even so, here are a few things to consider.

Simplify. It pays to choose simple foods rather than processed food products. The fewer ingredients, the better—one is ideal. Beans, broccoli, carrots, or brown rice, for example, do not need an ingredients list, because what you see is exactly what you get. You know that no one has added any oil or processed away any fiber.

Add more raw foods. Some people have had remarkable weight loss as a result of increasing their intake of raw foods. Chopped vegetables, salads, fresh fruit—these are all rich in fiber, with no added fat and low GIs.

BLOOD GLUCOSE NOT COMING UNDER CONTROL QUICKLY ENOUGH

The primary way of tracking your glucose control is with hemoglobin A1C. As you know, the American Diabetes Association's goal is to have your A1C under 7.0 percent. If you are not making good progress toward your goal, here are some points to consider.

Get back to the basics (again). If you are overweight, weight loss is the strongest predictor of a healthy drop in A1C. To jump-start weight loss, take a look at the tips above and in Chapter 6. Whether you are overweight or not, those same points are also the keys to bringing your glucose under control.

If your diet is vegan, it has no animal fat in it, of course. And if you are setting aside vegetable oils, it has very little of any kind of fat. With these healthy changes, you can just imagine those little bits of fat inside your muscle cells starting to shrivel up. As you saw in Chapter 2, these are the bits of fat that appear to be the cause of insulin resistance.

Embrace healthy carbohydrates. Many people tie one arm behind their backs by avoiding starchy foods. They imagine that beans, lentils, pasta, sweet potatoes, or yams will push their blood glucose upward. And, of course, if you check your blood glucose after just about any meal, it will be higher than it was before. However, don't let this turn you against starchy foods and back toward fatty or high-protein foods. Here is why.

The fat in fish and chicken will tend to arrest your weight loss. It will also tend to aggravate your insulin resistance. Here is what happens in a typical case.

A man has heard that "carbs are bad" or perhaps notices that his blood glucose has gone up briefly after a meal of rice or starchy vegetables. He decides to avoid carbohydrates and adds fish and chicken back into his diet. At first, it seems like a good change. His blood glucose does not spike strongly after meals because there is very little starch in his meals to provide glucose. "Aha!" he says. "I've found the diet to keep my blood sugar down!" Over the next several days, however, he notices that his fasting blood glucose values are heading in the wrong direction. They go up bit by bit, and after a week or two, the rise is significant. "Now what?" he thinks. This is what is going on:

There are only three sources of calories: carbohydrate, fat, and protein. In avoiding carbohydrate, he was left with fat—which tends to increase insulin resistance—and protein, which has problems of its own. The increased fat intake did not increase his blood glucose immediately, but fatty diets tend to increase the amount of fat inside the cells. The result is that insulin resistance gradually worsens. This means that any carbohydrate he ate later would cause a bigger blood sugar spike than it otherwise would have. As the days went by, his blood sugar gradually increased.

The answer to this is to avoid fatty foods and choose healthy, carbohydrate-rich foods, letting the glycemic index help you choose the best of them (see Chapter 4). This means legumes (beans, peas, and lentils), vegetables, fruits, and whole grains.

Meals will always cause a temporary rise in blood glucose; what you are looking for is an overall trend downward as your insulin sensitivity gradually improves.

See your doctor. One common reason for rising blood glucose levels is infection. A cold, a urinary tract infection, a foot sore, an ear infection—you name it. They all tend to raise your blood glucose.

Sometimes a surprisingly small cut or a cough you're hardly aware of boosts your fasting blood sugar values. As the infection heals (with medical treatment as needed), your blood glucose will recover. Your doctor may decide to adjust your diabetes medications in the interim.

Check your stress level. Stress raises blood sugar. The fight-or-flight response—the physical reaction that gets you ready to fight or run away from danger—can kick in with any sort of threat, real or imagined. A rise in blood sugar was much more useful when the threats we encountered were predators and warring tribes. That extra blood sugar fueled the muscles needed to run or fight. Today, we are more likely to be threatened by job worries, financial difficulties, or relationship problems, and rising blood sugar doesn't help during those times. But stress still evokes the response, and it still causes a blood sugar spike.

If stress is temporary, you will see your glucose spike resolve quickly. If stress is ongoing, get help. Meditation, yoga, and other techniques can help you deal with stress. If the problem is deeper—if you are headed into depression or chronic anxiety—do not try to be a hero. See a qualified mental health professional and get started with a treatment that works for you.

Exercise. If you are sedentary, now is the time to bring physical activity into your life. Vigorous exercise helps reduce blood glucose levels. See Chapter 11.

In most cases, these steps will help bring your blood sugar down. If it remains high despite your best efforts, your doctor will want to adjust your medications.

PERSISTENT HUNGER

If you are cutting back on calories in an effort to lose weight, you may be left feeling hungry. One of the reasons I recommend a low-fat, vegan diet is that it is so substantial—it provides plenty of fiber to fill you up and has no limits on portion sizes or calories. The result is weight loss without hunger. In our research studies, we use a questionnaire to measure hunger along the way, and we consistently find that this way of eating leaves people feeling satisfied.

What if your meals don't quite hold you, though? Here are some suggestions, starting with the obvious one.

Eat more. Maybe that little bowl of oatmeal is just not enough. When you are just getting to know new foods, it takes a little time to figure out the right serving sizes. You will soon sort this out.

Go low GI and high fiber. If you have instant oatmeal for breakfast, you will get hungry sooner than if you have the old-fashioned variety. The difference is simply that instant oats have had their fiber sliced up. Instead of flat rolled oats, you have a box full of oat powder. That means that they cook quicker but also that they digest quicker, spike your blood sugar quicker (that is, they have a higher GI), and leave you hungry quicker. Eating foods that are in as natural a state as possible prevents that overly rapid digestion and helps keep hunger at bay.

You want foods that have both a low GI *and* high fiber content. A food that offers one doesn't necessarily have the other. For example, whole wheat bread has lots of fiber, but something about the wheat grain causes it to release its natural sugars into the bloodstream rather quickly (i.e., it has a high GI). In fact, white bread (which has had its fiber removed) has virtually the same GI as whole wheat. In contrast, rye bread digests more slowly, releasing its natural sugars into the bloodstream more gradually, which means it has a low GI. To check your fiber intake, do a Quick Fiber Check (see page 112).

Have healthy snacks. There will be many times when you will want to have a bite to eat between meals, and you should! See Chapter 5 for a discussion of the best choices.

QUIETING CRAVINGS

If you have had diabetes for any length of time, you have already been coping with the ubiquitous nature of junk food. Unhealthy snacks are everywhere. But why do they call to us as they do? Why is sugar or chocolate sometimes so attractive? Why is cheese or meat sometimes hard to resist? Where do cravings come from?

One of our research participants once asked me what was wrong with her. She had had diabetes for 12 years, and even though she knew that she should stay away from sugary foods, she craved them. Especially when she was stressed or tired, cookies, chocolate, and pastries seemed to call her name. She had the cravings nearly every day. "I think I'm just a weak-willed person," she said. She was embarrassed about her cravings and found herself avoiding the subject when she spoke to her dietitian.

Here is the most important thing to understand about cravings: They are not caused by weak will or gluttony. Cravings are triggered by *biological properties of the foods themselves*. That is, certain foods have chemical makeups that cause us to crave them in very much the same way that drugs, alcohol, and tobacco have addictive components.

Let me be clear: Only certain foods lend themselves to cravings. The same foods are alluring to almost everyone.

Four types of foods trigger biochemical effects not unlike those of addictive drugs. They are not as strong or as dangerous as drugs, but the chemistry of addiction does seem to be at work with these foods. I have described these effects in detail in a book called *Breaking the Food Seduction*. Here, I will summarize the main points you need to know. The four categories of addictive food are sugar, chocolate, cheese, and meat.

Sugar. Sugar is not simply sweet. In addition to its taste, it also has a mild druglike effect. That is, it affects the brain in essentially the same way as opiate drugs—morphine and heroin, for example—albeit not as strongly. This effect helps explain why people crave sugar, especially during times of stress.

How do we know that sugar has this effect? In controlled studies, researchers use a medication called naloxone as a research tool. Naloxone is normally used in emergency rooms to block the effects of heroin or other opiates. If a person has overdosed on heroin, doctors inject naloxone, which blocks the heroin (and any other narcotic) from attaching to receptors in the brain. A comatose drug addict, previously on the verge of death, rapidly awakens with a dose of naloxone.

Researchers have given naloxone to volunteers and offered them various sugary foods. They then measured how much the volunteers ate and compared the results to those of the same test done without naloxone.

It turns out that naloxone causes a noticeable drop in sugar cravings. Normally, you might long for a glazed doughnut or piece of pie, but with a dose of naloxone, much of the attraction is gone. The effect is particularly clear for foods that contain both sugar and fat: cookies, cakes, and ice cream.

Naloxone is given intravenously and is not a treatment for food addiction; it is a research tool. These experiments show that sugar does not simply delight the taste buds; it also stimulates the release of opiate chemicals in the brain. Just as intense exercise causes the release of endorphins—natural feel-good chemicals within the brain—sugar seems to do something very similar.

Let me be clear about this: Sugar does not contain opiates. Rather, the taste of sugar on the tongue is what apparently triggers the release of opiates within the brain. In turn, these opiates trigger the release of another natural chemical, called dopamine, which is the key to the brain's pleasure centers. Drugs of abuse—heroin, cocaine, marijuana, tobacco, alcohol, and all others—increase dopamine activity in the brain. Sugar appears to do the same. Evidence suggests that the effects of sugar on the brain ease pain and discomfort and give us a little boost. No wonder we turn to sugary foods, especially when we're stressed.

Sugar has the same effects on infants just a few hours old. When babies have a heel-stick to draw a blood sample, they cry noticeably less if a bit of sugar water is dribbled into their mouth first.

Sugar cravings go beyond plain sugar itself. Some people also crave foods such as white bread or bagels, which turn to sugar rapidly and release sugar into the bloodstream. In essence, they crave high-GI foods—sugar, cookies, crackers, white bread, potatoes, or cold cereals. While we also enjoy low-GI foods, we tend not to crave them.

Chocolate. Chocolate's addictive qualities have long been recognized in psychiatric journals. And in scientific studies, the most ardent chocoholics' desire falls away when they are treated with opiate-blocking drugs. These experiments show that it is not simply taste or mouthfeel that keeps us hooked. Chocolate also appears to have mild effects on our brains.

Chocolate's attraction is not due simply to its sweetness. After all, no true chocolate lover would be satisfied with sugar alone. Chocolate also contains caffeine, theobromine, and phenylethylamine. These are all stimulants, and they may play a role in chocolate's seduction, aside from its opiate effects.

If you are a chocolate lover, you probably already know that chocolate is more than a food: You don't just feel you *want* it, you feel you *need it*. Regrettably, chocolate carries not only a load of sugar but also a considerable load of fat.

Cheese. Yes, it may smell a bit like old socks, but cheese is one of the foods that people who are trying to improve their diets have the most trouble leaving behind. There is obviously something besides fat and cholesterol in cheese that accounts for its popularity.

That "something" may be the dairy protein, or casein. Like all proteins, casein's molecular structure is like a long string of beads, with each bead being an amino acid. Normally, when proteins are digested, these amino acids come apart one by one and are absorbed into the bloodstream to be used to build body tissues and repair any damage to your body.

Casein behaves differently. As it breaks apart, it does not simply release individual amino acids. It breaks into short strings of amino acids—strings of perhaps four, five, or seven "beads." They are not just the amino acid building blocks for protein; they are also biologically active compounds with a mild narcotic action. Scientists call them casomorphins—casein-derived morphinelike compounds. If scientists were to feed you cheese and then take a sample of your digestive tract contents, they would find an array of casomorphins with mild narcotic actions. Some have speculated that the narcotic effects of casomorphins are responsible for cheese's attraction. These effects may also explain why cheese can be constipating, since narcotic compounds slow digestion.

By now you know if cheese is your thing. If so, its fat and cholesterol contents are conspiring against you. Shortly, we will look at how to kick this and other food addictions.

Meat. Men, in particular, often describe meat as the very last food they would ever want to give up. No matter how often they are reminded of what it is doing to their waistline or cholesterol test results, many have trouble breaking their emotional attachment to roast beef, steak, or chicken wings.

Once again, experiments with opiate-blocking drugs suggest that part of the desire for meat may have its basis in opiate effects within the brain. Researchers in England gave opiate-blocking drugs to volunteers and tested their desire for ham, salami, and tuna. The results showed that when the opiate effects were blocked, volunteers lost much of their interest in meat.[1]

RESETTING YOUR PRIORITIES

If cravings are sabotaging your new food program, take heart. You are not the victim of a bad upbringing or a gluttonous personality. The fact is, you are not attracted to just any food, or even to most foods. You may like apples, oranges, bananas, or asparagus, but you have never once turned to them for solace during moments of stress. You have never raced off to a convenience store because you just *had* to have cauliflower. You have turned to sugar, chocolate, cheese, or meat because they have chemical effects on the brain. Some beverages, such as wine or coffee, also have druglike effects and can be addictive. But as far as foods go, those four are the ones that work their unfortunate magic on just about everyone.

Before we see what you might eat instead of that sugary doughnut, candy bar, or cheeseburger, let's take a closer look at what happens inside your brain when you eat these foods.

A network of cells deep inside the brain makes up what is sometimes called your reward center. Indeed, it is responsible for feelings of pleasure. Without it, life would be one big gray day.

The reward center is not there just for fun, however. It is there to keep you alive and to maintain the species. Here is why: If you got absolutely no pleasure from eating, you might forget about foods entirely! Likewise, if sex were a total bore, the species would soon die out. Thus, when you eat or have sex, your reward center gives you a little bit of dopamine as a kind of reward.

In the process, that dopamine release causes slight neurological changes, changes that put high-priority status on repeating whatever you have just done. "That was fun," your reward center seems to say. "Let's be sure to do that again."

In nature, this would mean getting a reward for finding a new food source or a receptive mate, with the result that you would take advantage of your find again and again. The problem is that this system is easily hijacked. Alcohol, recreational drugs, tobacco—and yes, unhealthy foods—cause significant dopamine release, so not only do you like them, you also want to have them again and again. Your pleasure center rearranges your priorities to favor whatever stimulated it most recently. You find yourself planning your day around sugar or chocolate, just as an alcoholic might regularly think about where the next drink is coming from. If you have ever wondered why these otherwise banal foods have such sway, it is because they hijack your brain's pleasure circuitry and your internal priority-setting system.

Breaking Free

If the occasional taste of sugar or chocolate is really not a big part of your life, there is no need to worry about it. But if your waistline is expanding before your very eyes, or your health is suffering from your food habits, it is time to wake up and smell the addiction. What do you do if you're hooked?

The best way to deal with unhealthy foods is to avoid teasing yourself. Set them aside completely, at least for now. Do not keep them in the house, and do not buy them. There is no need to worry about whether you will return to them in the future. For now, just leave them alone.

In the process, your brain's priorities can return to what really is good for you. You are likely to find that your desire for unhealthy foods fades the longer you are away from them. The following steps will also help.

- Eat a healthy breakfast, and don't skip meals. Cravings kick in when you are hungry.

- Get regular exercise so you're tired enough to sleep soundly, and be sure to get plenty of rest. Cravings are stronger when you are not sleeping well.

- Avoid situations that trigger cravings. Some people find that their cravings are triggered by being alone, by television cooking shows, by concession stands at movie theaters, or by certain friends who are preoccupied with food problems of their own. Try to identify your triggers and eliminate them as much as possible.

Getting the Taste without the Regrets

Sometimes a simple substitution can help you steer away from an unhealthful food. Here are a few.

If you crave sugar: In recipes, maple syrup, molasses, sorghum syrup, and granulated sugarcane juice (Sucanat) can sometimes substitute for table sugar. These are hardly health foods! But the idea is to replace refined white sugar with a smaller amount of syrup or juice. They're so flavorful you won't notice you're using less.

Stevia is an intensely sweet derivative of an herb from Paraguay. It is sold as a dietary supplement (its use as a commercial food additive has not yet been approved).

Sucralose (Splenda) is a calorie-free sweetener made from cane sugar to which chlorine has been chemically added, greatly increasing the sweetness of the final product. Sugar alcohols, such as mannitol, sorbitol, and xylitol, are low-calorie sweeteners sometimes used in candies, chewing gum, and desserts. They have about half the calories of table sugar. There are, of course, other artificial sweeteners. The disadvantage of the lot of them is that they do not help you break your love affair with sweets, so when artificial sweeteners are not available, you will find yourself returning to sugar.

My friend and colleague Hans Diehl, DrHSc, founder of the Coronary Health Improvement Project, says the best thing to do for a sweet tooth is to "have it pulled!" The idea is that if you set sweets aside, you will eventually just forget about them.

Of course, the best choices are fresh fruits—nature's sweet foods. It also helps to make sure your diet has adequate complex carbohydrate—grains, sweet potatoes, and beans, for example. These foods provide the energy you need in a form that is much more healthful than sugar.

If you crave chocolate: Cocoa powder is essentially defatted chocolate. It can be used in beverages and baking or turned into a dip for strawberries or other fresh fruit. You can also find low-fat frozen ice cream substitutes made from soy, as well as sorbets.

If you crave cheese: Get to know nutritional yeast. Sold in the supplement aisle of health food stores, nutritional yeast flakes (not brewer's or baker's yeast) add a cheeselike flavor to sauces and casseroles.

In recipes, you can replace ricotta or cottage cheese with mashed, water-packed tofu mixed with a little lemon juice. If you're choosing soy cheeses, read the label to check the fat content and to see whether they're made with added casein, the dairy protein.

If you crave meat: Good substitutes for hot dogs, burgers, and deli meats are now widely available. Seitan (made from wheat gluten), tofu, tempeh, and textured vegetable protein are versatile products that substitute well for meat in recipes. Surprisingly enough, the desire for meat fades very rapidly once it is removed from the diet. People who thought they could not live without steak or a salmon fillet soon find they have absolutely no desire for it.

Genetic Influences on Cravings

Although cravings can affect anyone, some people may be especially vulnerable. Researchers have found that some people are born with fewer receptors for dopamine, the brain chemical responsible for pleasurable feelings. Apparently, this lack of receptors means that they get less dopamine stimulation and less of the feel-good sensation that dopamine provides. This leaves them feeling a bit out of sorts compared with other people. As a result, they are drawn to tobacco, alcohol, or drugs; presumably, they are seeking the stimulation that nature has not given them. They may even fall prey to compulsive gambling or compulsive eating.

It all starts with a gene. The receptors for dopamine are built according to the specifications on your chromosomes—the long spiral staircase–shaped strings of genes in each of your cells that determine who you are. Your mother and father passed along their genes to you, and the makeup of your body reflects the combination of the two. If either parent passed along a gene for having too few dopamine receptors,

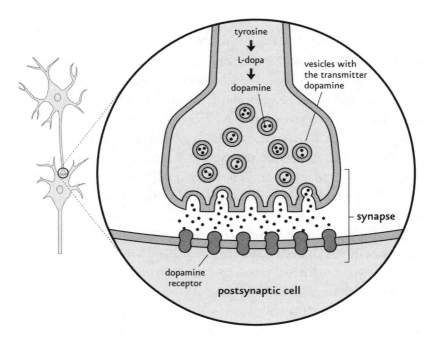

The brain cell at the top contains small packets (vesicles) of dopamine. When you experience a pleasurable sensation, these vesicles release their dopamine into the space (synapse) that lies between that cell and the next one. As the dopamine molecules reach the next cell, they attach to its dopamine receptors, and their effect depends on how many dopamine receptors you have. Some people have approximately one-third fewer receptors than other people.

you would have roughly one-third fewer receptors than other people.

If you were able to sample individuals in smoking cessation programs or drug treatment clinics, you would find that as many as 40 percent have a gene that causes them to have too few receptors, called dopamine receptor D2, or DRD2 for short.

Several years ago, I found myself wondering if people who have trouble following a healthful diet may have this genetic variation. Ernest Noble, MD, of the University of California, Los Angeles, conducted genetic analyses on our patients. To our surprise, we found that nearly half of our research participants with type 2 diabetes had the gene that was associated with fewer than normal dopamine receptors. That is far higher than the roughly one-in-five prevalence in the general population.

This raised a disturbing question: Did the lack of dopamine receptors lead them to overeat? Did overeating then lead to weight gain, which in turn triggered diabetes? We have not yet sorted all this out, but we did find that while people with this gene improved a great deal on our diet, they got somewhat less benefit compared to those with the normal number of dopamine receptors. Their A1C values dropped by about 0.9 percentage point on average, compared to a drop of 1.6 points for those without the gene. At present, this type of genetic testing is done only in research studies. Your doctor cannot determine whether you are genetically endowed with fewer dopamine receptors. In fact, as far as your food plan is concerned, it does not matter. Regardless of your genetic makeup, the diet described in this book is very likely to help you. I raise the issue of genetics simply to underscore the point that cravings and food addictions are *physical*, not moral issues. They are due to the properties of foods themselves that interact with our natural biochemistry.

One final point: If certain foods act like drugs, it pays to treat them like drugs. In other words, avoid them. Just as it is harder for a smoker to cut down than to quit and harder for an alcoholic to drink wine moderately than to quit drinking altogether, it is very tough to tease yourself with foods that have you in their clutches. It is actually easier to leave them alone completely and do your best to forget about them. If you have not had one of these biochemically active foods in a few weeks, you crave it much less than you would if you had it yesterday.

DIGESTIVE PROBLEMS

A plant-based diet is great for people who have been bothered by constipation. Its natural fiber is what your digestive tract needs. Some foods can cause a bit of gassiness, however. If you experience this, here is what to do about it.

First, only certain foods cause gas. Grains, fruits, and most vegetables get a not-guilty verdict. Beans and undercooked cruciferous vegetables (broccoli, cabbage, cauliflower, and Brussels sprouts, for example) are the main culprits. Chances are, all you need to do is have smaller servings. If you have been replacing a huge steak with a huge plate of beans, remember that a small amount of beans goes a long way. Try downsizing your portions.

Over time, you will find that your body adjusts, so you can have larger portions with less gassiness. If you cook beans from scratch, be sure to discard the water used to soak them and then cook them in fresh water. Cook them well (there are no *al dente* beans)! The same goes for cruciferous vegetables. Yes, we all love a stalk of fresh broccoli from the crudités tray, but if that gives you digestive trouble, cook vegetables until you can easily pierce them with a fork.

It goes without saying that you want to avoid dairy products and sugar. Dairy products, of course, are already off the list, but digestive problems are yet another reason to steer clear of them, as you saw in Chapter 4. The lactose (milk sugar) that makes up fully 55 percent of the calories in fat-free milk causes many people to have gas, cramps, and diarrhea. Here is why.

During infancy, the lactase enzyme is produced within the body and breaks lactose apart in the baby's intestinal tract so it can be absorbed and used for energy. As children leave infancy behind, however, most lose this enzyme. The result, lactose intolerance, was once thought to be abnormal, but it is now known to be the biological norm, not only for humans but for all mammals. Because the body's lactase production slacks off gradually, many people do not make the connection between their digestive symptoms and milk products.

In about 85 percent of Caucasians, a genetic mutation causes the lactase enzyme to persist well into adulthood. Even so, lactose intolerance will eventually affect many of them, too. Deleting dairy products from the menu for a few days will show you whether you are among them.

Some adults have trouble digesting table sugar (sucrose). Once again, it is easy to check. Simply set it aside for a few days and see if your symptoms improve.

HIGH TRIGLYCERIDES

When your doctor checks your cholesterol, triglycerides will also be listed on the laboratory report. Triglycerides are molecules of fat that are transported in the blood for various purposes. As with cholesterol, having a certain amount of triglycerides in the blood is a normal part of human biochemistry. However, when triglycerides are high, they increase the risk of heart problems, diseases of the pancreas, and other problems. As you saw in Chapter 7, a normal triglyceride concentration is less than 150 mg/dl. Values of 150 to 199 mg/dl are considered borderline, and values of 200 to 499 mg/dl are high. Concentrations of 500 mg/dl or higher are considered very high.

Some studies have suggested that diets high in refined carbohydrates may cause a temporary rise in triglycerides. High-fiber and low-GI foods appear to have the opposite effect.[2] You will want to make a special point of favoring these foods. In our research, a low-fat, low-GI, vegan diet brings down triglyceride levels very effectively. In addition, a low-fat, vegan diet helps you lose weight, which in turn reduces triglycerides.

Regular exercise helps, too. Moderate physical activity, such as walking, lowers triglyceride concentrations. You will also benefit by avoiding alcohol. Alcohol appears to raise triglycerides slightly, so when you avoid it, triglycerides slide back down.

INTERACTION BETWEEN VEGETABLES AND PRESCRIPTION BLOOD THINNERS

Warfarin (Coumadin) is a blood thinner prescribed to prevent heart attacks, strokes, blood clots in the legs, and other problems. It acts by antagonizing the effects of vitamin K, which is involved in building the proteins your body uses in the clotting process.

Many people taking warfarin believe they have to avoid vegetables, especially green leafy vegetables, that are rich in vitamin K because the vitamin will affect their tendency to form clots. But avoiding these healthful foods would leave them very low in important vitamins and minerals.

I encourage you to discuss this issue with your doctor and your dietitian, but the answer is not to avoid vegetables. What matters is maintaining a fairly steady amount of them in your diet so your warfarin dosage does not need to be continually adjusted. If you eat lots of healthy vegetables and then suddenly stop, warfarin's actions become stronger, increasing the risk of bleeding. On the other hand, if you were to generally avoid vegetables and one day suddenly increase your intake, the vitamin K in these foods would have the opposite effect, making it easier for your body to form clots. Bottom line: Enjoy vegetables and keep the amount fairly constant from day to day.

By the way, alcohol increases warfarin's effects, which is why doctors encourage people taking it to avoid alcohol. Many medications (e.g., aspirin, acetaminophen, and many others) can also accentuate warfarin's action.

If you have hit any bumps in the road, I hope you have found these suggestions helpful and that you are now back on track with a healthful diet.

CHAPTER 10

Which Supplements Should You Take?

News stories and advertisements trumpet the benefits of various nutritional supplements. Drugstores and health food shops are stocked with shelf after shelf of them. Which ones help, and which ones are unnecessary?

Here is some basic information that will help you decide. You should, however, talk to your doctor, nurse practitioner, pharmacist, or dietitian about which products you may take. You may have a particular need for one or another supplement depending on your health. Or you may need to avoid certain products because they interfere with medications you are taking.

If you are adding supplements that might affect your blood sugar, be sure to check your blood glucose regularly. Refer to Chapter 7 for how to recognize and treat low blood sugar.

Let's look at specific vitamins and other nutritional compounds, starting with the basics.

Vitamin B_{12}. This vitamin is essential for healthy blood cells and nerve function. If you follow a vegan diet, as I recommend, you should take a daily vitamin B_{12} supplement that provides at least 5 micrograms. Nearly all brands contain more than this, but higher doses are not toxic. Many people, particularly older people, tend to run low on vitamin B_{12} regardless of their diets, because their bodies become less efficient at absorbing it. That is also true of people taking metformin or acid-blocking medications. Yes, you can find vitamin B_{12} in some fortified products, such as breakfast cereals and soy milk, but the amounts may not be enough to meet your needs.

Vitamin D. Vitamin D is produced when your skin is exposed to sunlight. It helps you absorb calcium, among other functions. It is a good idea to spend 15 to 20 minutes daily outdoors. If you get this sun exposure, there is no need for dietary supplementation. If you do not and also do not take a regular multivitamin, a 2,000 IU vitamin D supplement is a good idea.

Aside from the basic vitamins, some other supplements have shown promise for people with diabetes.

Cinnamon. Cinnamon has been shown to improve blood sugar levels. As little as ½ teaspoon of ordinary cinnamon added to your morning oatmeal or other foods not only seems to reduce blood sugar, but also appears to reduce blood cholesterol levels.[1] Some of cinnamon's helpful effects may be explained by compounds called polyphenol polymers, which are found in the spice and have an insulin-like action.

Magnesium. In Harvard's Nurses' Health Study, women who had more magnesium in their diets had a significantly lower likelihood of developing diabetes.[2] Apparently, magnesium increases insulin sensitivity and may increase the secretion of insulin from the pancreas, which suggests that it may also be helpful after diabetes has been diagnosed.

This does not mean, however, that you need a magnesium supplement. Foods rich in magnesium include whole grains (grains with their natural fiber intact) such as brown rice, barley, and oats, as well as green vegetables such as spinach and Swiss chard. Many bean varieties are also rich in magnesium.

Chromium. Chromium is an element that helps insulin work better, meaning that it helps the hormone escort glucose from your bloodstream into your cells.

Technically speaking, chromium is what is called an insulin cofactor—an insulin helper, if you will. In the same way that you cannot use a jack to lift your car if its handle is missing, insulin has trouble bringing glucose into cells without chromium to help it work properly.

Chromium's essential role was discovered only relatively recently. In the late 1960s, researchers found that chromium deficiency could lead to high blood sugar levels.[3] In 1977, Canadian researchers described the case of a woman in her midthirties who was receiving all her nutrition intravenously following intestinal surgery. As time went by, she began to lose weight. Her blood sugar started to rise inexplicably, and eventually, she developed nerve symptoms in her legs that appeared to be diabetic neuropathy. Her doctors had to administer large insulin doses to bring her blood sugar under control. Eventually, they gave her chromium, which had been absent from her feeding formula. In just a few weeks, her blood glucose fell to the point where she no longer required insulin, and her nerve symptoms disappeared.[4]

Chromium is naturally present in many foods, such as broccoli, green beans, whole grains, nuts, and even coffee. Some experts recommend taking supplements as well.

Which foods have it, and how much do we need? According to the Food and Nutrition Board of the Institute of Medicine, the safe and adequate daily intakes of chromium for adults ages 19 to 50 are 35 micrograms for men and 25 micrograms for women. For people over 50, the amounts are 30 micrograms for men and 20 micrograms for women. Here is the amount of chromium in common foods, as listed by the US government.

Chromium Content of Common Foods		
FOOD	PORTION	CHROMIUM (MCG)
Broccoli	½ cup, cooked	11
Grape juice	1 cup	8
English muffin, whole wheat	1	4
Potatoes, mashed	1 cup, cooked	3
Garlic, dried	1 teaspoon	3
Basil, dried	1 tablespoon	2
Orange juice	1 cup	2
Whole wheat bread	2 slices	2
Red wine	5 ounces	1–13
Apple, with skin	1 medium	1
Banana	1 medium	1
Green beans	½ cup, cooked	1

Source: National Institutes of Health, http://ods.od.nih.gov/factsheets/Chromium_pf.asp#h2, accessed April 10, 2017.

While you are making sure to include chromium-rich foods in your menu, it may also help to steer clear of sugar and refined grain products such as white flour. These foods are not only low in chromium, they also increase chromium loss from the body. Loss of the mineral is also increased by the stresses of infection, strenuous exercise, and pregnancy.

Some researchers have gone beyond foods and have tested the effects of supplements. However, studies in which researchers gave chromium to people with type 1, type 2, or gestational diabetes have yielded mixed results. The problem may be that some studies were small and used rather small chromium doses, but some studies using higher doses in individuals with type 2 diabetes have shown no benefit.[5] As a result, most diabetes authorities do not recommend chromium supplements.

If you are going to supplement, you should be aware that the safety of high chromium doses has not been as extensively studied as that of other minerals. Studies using chromium for diabetes treatment often exceed the amounts recommended by the US government, using doses of up to 1,000 micrograms per day. Individuals with impaired liver or kidney function may be at risk for adverse effects and should probably stay well below this level. The long-term benefits and risks of chromium supplementation are not known.

Alpha-lipoic acid. Alpha-lipoic acid, sometimes called thioctic acid, is naturally produced in the human body. It plays important roles in the mitochondria, the microscopic "burners" that provide energy in the cells. It works as a cofactor for several enzymes related to energy metabolism.

Supplemental alpha-lipoic acid is used not to counteract deficiencies but to act essentially like a drug. In high doses, it acts as an antioxidant. In people with type 2 diabetes, it appears to increase insulin sensitivity and reduce symptoms of nerve damage.[6, 7]

In many studies of alpha-lipoic acid, researchers used intravenous infusions rather than oral doses. So far, it appears to be safe, but it is not yet clear whether it will yield clinically important effects over the long run and if so, what doses are safe and effective for long-term use.

For Further Reference

If you search for information about supplements on the Web, you may find yourself carried away by a flood of commercial sites. I recommend this National Institutes of Health site, cc.nih.gov/ccc/supplements.

CHAPTER 11

Exercise for the Rest of Us

Yes, exercise is good for you. Physical activity reduces your blood sugar and is good for your heart. It improves the quality of your sleep and your overall energy level. When you get into an exercise groove, you really feel great.

For many of us, however, exercise conjures up images of painful workouts and unrewarding drudgery. Many people have trouble getting into an exercise routine; it just does not seem to work for them. For every person I hear say something like this:

> "I feel so good when I exercise. I have more energy, my blood sugar comes way down, and I just feel great. I can't imagine a day without it."

. . . there's another who feels more like this:

> "I really just can't get into exercise. I know I'd do better if I did, but every time I join a gym or resolve to start exercising, it just doesn't last."

If you are carrying around a lot of extra weight, exercise can be difficult. Perhaps you are limited by joint pain or heart problems. Maybe your good intentions just seem to vanish when the time comes to lace up your sneakers. In this chapter, we will tackle the various aspects of exercise—its benefits, its limitations, and the difficulties in getting started—and see how to make it work for you.

One note of reassurance: If you cannot exercise because of a physical limitation, you can still lose weight, cut your blood sugar, and live a healthy life. In fact, most of the benefits of the diet changes you have read about came *without* exercise. That is because in our diet studies, we usually ask our volunteers *not* to alter their exercise patterns, so we can isolate the effects of a diet change for research purposes. Exercise certainly adds to the health benefits that a good diet brings, but if it is simply not in the picture, you can still do well.

WHAT YOU ARE WORKING FOR

Different kinds of exercise provide very different benefits.

Aerobic exercise is any sort of rhythmic, continuous activity you perform for a sustained period—usually at least 10 minutes. Brisk walking, running, playing tennis, dancing, or skating can all be aerobic. This type of exercise reduces your blood sugar and triglycerides, and if you keep it up, you will live longer.

Resistance exercise is weight lifting and other exercises in which the emphasis is on muscular effort: pushups and deep knee bends, for example. It builds your muscle mass or at least preserves the muscle you have. It also improves insulin sensitivity.

Flexibility exercises (stretching) are intended to maintain the range of motion of your joints. They can also relieve stress.

Below, I will give you guidelines for how much and how often you should exercise.

A diet–exercise combination can help prevent diabetes from ever developing. A groundbreaking study called the Diabetes Prevention Program followed 3,234 people whose blood sugar levels were creeping upward but were not yet high enough to warrant a diagnosis of diabetes. With a combination of diet and exercise, the participants were able to cut the risk of developing the disease by 58 percent. The exercise regimen totaled 150 minutes per week—a half hour five times a week.[1]

There is a very big caveat with all of this, though: Exercise can boost the effects of a healthy diet, but it cannot make up for a poor one. In fact, of the two components—diet and exercise—the diet portion is much more important for weight loss and ultimately for preventing or controlling diabetes.

A careful review of published research showed that people who begin exercise programs do not lose much more weight than people who remain sedentary.[2] For weight control, exercise cannot take the place of diet changes.

This does not mean that exercise is of no help at all. It is definitely helpful for reducing A1C. In a review of several studies testing the effect of exercise, the average A1C in volunteers who began exercise programs fell to 7.7 percent, which is better than the 8.3 percent found in those who did not exercise.[3] Once again, however, that result pales in comparison to the benefits of a diet change. To prevent diabetes or bring it under control, it is best to use both diet *and* exercise.

One part of your body that benefits tremendously from exercise is your heart. A recent study tracked physical activity levels in adults with type 2 diabetes over a period of 19 years and looked specifically at the risk of dying of heart disease. It turned out that those who were moderately physically active were about 40 percent less likely to succumb to heart disease than were sedentary people. Their routines included at least 4 hours per week of moderate exercise such as walking, cycling, or light gardening.[4] Active people also cut their risk of stroke.[5]

There are three other exercise benefits worth noting. First, exercise and eating are mutually exclusive activities. It is easy to scarf down extra calories while watching your favorite crime drama or a movie, but it is a real challenge while you are playing tennis. Exercise is calorie-free fun.

Second, exercise helps you sleep. If you have given your muscles a good workout, they *demand* sleep. You will sleep much more soundly than if you had spent the entire day behind your desk, watching television, or reading. And when you are well rested, it is easier to stay focused on a healthy diet and say no to unhealthful foods.

Third, exercise makes you feel better. It lifts your spirits and is a natural antidepressant.

TYPE I AND TYPE II MUSCLE CELLS

Why do some people love exercise and others loathe it? Surprisingly enough, part of the reason is genetic. If you could look inside your muscles and compare them with those of other people, you would discover a sobering fact: Some people were born to exercise. That is to say, their muscles naturally contain many type I cells (the name has nothing to do with type 1 diabetes; it is just a coincidence). These muscle cells have a particularly strong blood supply made possible by a rich network of capillaries that bring in oxygen and reduce fatigue. They also have an extra supply of an enzyme called lipoprotein lipase, which breaks fats apart to be used as fuel. The result is extra energy for a long run. When you see people running down the road looking invigorated rather than haggard, or when someone waxes poetic about the joys of the runner's high, do not envy their resolve. Odds are, they were born with muscles that are just loaded with type I cells.

Other people's muscles contain mostly type II cells, which are fine for short bursts of exercise but have less endurance for the long haul.

Now, having said that, it is important to realize that muscles can change, at least to a degree. If you gradually but steadily increase the intensity of your workouts (within the limits of safety), the blood supply to type II cells increases. Eventually, they become almost as vigorous as type I cells.

I raise this biological distinction to make an important point: Exercise aptitude—or lack of it—is not a question of character; it is biology at work. If you have been beating yourself up for your lack of athletic prowess, it is time for a reprieve.

MAKING IT WORK FOR YOU

There are two keys to making exercise work.

First, let's keep it fun. For most of us, that means it should be a social event. It is more fun to go walking with someone else than by yourself. If you plan to exercise at a gym, you are much more likely to follow through if you sign up for a class—aerobics, yoga, or whatever—than if you go it alone. You are also much more likely to actually get to your class if someone is going with you.

You might make an occasion of it and plan an especially healthful meal afterward. If you are going dancing or playing tennis, the word *exercise* may not even enter your mind. Your activity is too enjoyable to call it that. Keep it fun because otherwise, you will not do it twice, much less three times a week. And for most people, fun means friends. You need other people with you to make it work.

Second, it is important to exercise regularly rather than intermittently. To paraphrase Newton's first law of motion, "an object at rest tends to stay at rest, and an object in motion tends to stay in motion." If the object at rest is you—that is, if you are firmly planted on the couch—you will tend to stay at rest. If, on the other hand, you and a friend go for a walk every other day after dinner, you will stay on track.

One important tip: As you get ready for an exercise session, you will have some misgivings. The little devil on your shoulder will tell you that you are too tired, you don't have time, you just don't feel like it, etc. But the fact is, you will *never* feel like it right at that "getting ready" moment. So don't wait for that perfect day when you will "feel like it." Just do it anyway, and do it now. Get on out there and do your thing. And very soon, you'll discover that you are glad you did.

This cycle will repeat itself every time you exercise—feelings of misgivings and negative thoughts, followed by your resolve to just ignore that negativity and do it anyway, followed by being so glad that you did. And before long, your confidence will grow and you'll get into a groove.

There is another reason for keeping exercise regular: The effect of any single exercise session is small. If you belong to a gym, you can see this for yourself. Just jump on the nearest treadmill and run flat out for a mile. Then, as you catch your breath, push the little button that lets you see how many calories you have burned. Surprised? That's right, you have expended only about 100 calories. That's less than half the calories in an order of McDonald's french fries or a bottle of soda. A single exercise session every now and then will not help you any more than occasionally eating a healthy meal. To be really effective, healthy habits have to be part of your routine.

Also, for better or worse, exercise effects do not last very long. If you are laid up with an injury, for example, you will find your blood sugar or weight gradually returning to its pre-exercise level. People who get into a habit of going for a brisk walk or bicycle ride every day or two sustain their benefits.

Bottom line: To make exercise work, keep it fun, and keep it regular.

SEE YOUR DOCTOR FIRST

Before you embark on a new exercise program, be sure to get your doctor's okay. Is your heart up to it? Are your joints ready? How vulnerable are you to hypo- or hyperglycemia? Do you have any special eye or foot problems that could be aggravated by exercise? Your doctor should address all of these questions.

Beware of jumping into vigorous exercise too quickly. If it has been months (or years) since you tried exercising regularly, start slowly. It takes time for your body to reap the rewards of your new, improved diet. A heart patient, for example, who begins a vegan diet, stops smoking, and starts really taking care of himself will probably feel better very soon. His chest pain may melt away within a few weeks, and he will be eager to jump into a vigorous exercise program. The fact is, though, that he still has the artery blockages he has been accumulating for years. Yes, the damage can be reversed, but it takes time, and he should not push himself past the limits set by his doctor.

If you have type 1 diabetes, you may find that your blood sugar drops precipitously during and after exercise. This can also happen to people with type 2 diabetes who use insulin or drugs that cause insulin secretion (e.g., glyburide, glipizide, glimepiride, nateglinide, or repaglinide). It is important to be alert to the possibility of a major blood sugar drop and to adjust your eating schedule, medication use, and exercise accordingly.

Occasionally, the opposite can occur: You may find that your blood sugar is temporarily higher after exercise than it was before.

A research team based in Florida tracked blood glucose in children with type 1 diabetes as they walked on a treadmill in four 15-minute bouts, with 5-minute rest periods in between. Their average blood glucose was 159 mg/dl when they started, and it fell to 112 mg/dl afterward. At least one-quarter of the children became hypoglycemic during or right after the exercise. They were also more likely to be hypoglycemic during the following night.[6]

Exercise can reduce your blood sugar surprisingly quickly. Of course, if you eat too much in an effort to prevent hypoglycemia, your blood sugar can go too high.

For these reasons, it is important to speak with your caregiver about your medication, diet, and exercise program to make sure you are ready for exercise, then make whatever adjustments are needed for safety.

GETTING STARTED

Okay. Your doctor has given you the green light, you have rustled up some friends, and you are ready to begin.

If you were imagining that I would push you into hours of jogging and weight lifting and harangue you with exhortations about "no pain, no gain"—well, push those thoughts aside. The goal is to enjoy exercise—so much so that it becomes part of your life.

For aerobic exercise, I suggest starting with a half-hour brisk walk 5 days a week, assuming that you have no health-related exercise restrictions. If you prefer, you can exercise three times per week, either taking brisk 1-hour walks or doing more vigorous half-hour workouts. You can also break up those 30-minute walks into 10- or 15-minute mini-workouts if you like. Do not allow yourself more than 2 sedentary days in a row. The benefits of walking are not as great as those of a more vigorous exercise program, but it is a good place to start.

The important thing is to find a time that works for you.

It is a good idea to put exercise on your schedule, as if it were an appointment with yourself, and to include someone else in your plans.

A pedometer will help you keep track of your progress. In our research studies, we use an Omron pedometer to track the total number of steps participants take each day as well as the number of "aerobic steps" (steps taken as part of a continuous walk of at least 10 minutes).

The participants can also program in their stride length to track mileage and even estimate their calorie burn. Take note of how many (or how few!) steps you take in a normal day, then gradually increase them. For reference, 10,000 steps or more is a vigorous day for a healthy person, but you may not have the strength or stamina to do that many. Do not push beyond your doctor's recommended limits.

A podiatrist or nurse specializing in diabetes (certified diabetes educator, or CDE) will help you take care of your feet. This is important since exercise can sometimes cause foot injuries or aggravate an existing injury. It is surprising how often people are unaware of gradually worsening foot sores.

Your doctor will help you gauge your improvement and can advise you about increasing your exercise intensity. As your endurance improves, you will find that your energy just keeps increasing, and your weight and blood sugar stay under better control.

What's Your Pleasure?

Taking a regular walk is a great way to start exercising. When you are ready to add other activities, think about which ones you might enjoy.

- Aerobics classes can be fun, social, and sometimes intense.
- Dancing is wonderful exercise, with better music than most aerobics classes.
- Tennis, either singles or doubles, can be a great workout.
- Many health clubs organize racquetball or handball lessons and competitions.
- Golf can be great exercise if you walk the course.
- Local running clubs often organize training groups for people working toward 5-K, 10-K, and half- and full-marathon races.

For resistance and flexibility exercises, I suggest that you work with a personal trainer, both for safety reasons and to individualize your program using the right equipment. Professional athletes are not the only ones with access to professional fitness expertise; you can have it, too. A personal trainer can help you plan a full program, not only for aerobics but also for strength training and flexibility.

Most health clubs have trainers on staff and may even offer a free session as an incentive to join. Why not take advantage of it? If you do not plan on joining a gym, just make an appointment for a single exercise counseling session so you can get a program that is right for you. Then schedule a follow-up.

No Blame, No Shame

With exercise, just as with diet, most people are not yet where they would like to be. Guilt and blame come into the picture when we are sedentary, just as they do when we are not eating well. Sometimes family members try to scold us into exercising, and sometimes doctors try the same approach. But all their moralizing is nothing compared to the guilt-laden punishment we heap on ourselves, as if not exercising were a tremendous moral failing.

If that is where you are, let me encourage you to set guilt and blame aside. Just let it all go. Tell your guilt-inducing friends that up until now, you have been illustrating Newton's first law of motion. Now, however, you are about to get into gear and explore the second part of that principle.

The same applies if you happen to fall off the wagon. Let's say you have let your exercise regimen lapse for a bit—maybe even a very long bit. Do not waste your time feeling bad about it; it happens to everybody. Just dust yourself off and get back on.

When exercise is fun and your friends or family are part of it—and when you start at a level that's right for you and keep it regular—you have the formula for success.

PART 3

Complete Health

CHAPTER 12

A Healthy Heart

Managing or reversing the effects of diabetes means more than getting your blood sugar under control. It also means regaining your health as much as you possibly can, and safeguarding it.

If you have been in poor health—or if diabetes has attacked your heart, eyes, kidneys, and nerves—revamping your diet can have a dramatic positive effect on your well-being. In this chapter and the next, we will look at how to keep your heart—and the rest of you—healthy.

TAKING RISK SERIOUSLY

You probably already have a good idea of your risk of heart problems. Your doctor has sized up your cholesterol level and blood pressure, and you know your family history. You may be on medications to control cholesterol or strengthen your heart.

The next step is to review what you need to know about risks, and more important, to see what you can do to prevent heart disease and, if necessary, reverse the disease process.

In evaluating your risk of developing heart problems, doctors look at your age, family history, smoking habits, weight, cholesterol level, blood pressure, and other factors. I believe, however, that it is prudent to *act* as if you are at risk even if none of these factors apply to you. Here is why: Most people in North America and Europe have already developed artery blockages—the beginnings of heart disease—by the time they reach early adulthood. Having diabetes increases that risk. Rather than wondering, "Am I at risk?" it is safe to simply assume that you are—and to take action to protect yourself.

Some evidence suggests that your heart is assaulted especially hard by smoking, high blood pressure, and high cholesterol levels, while your small blood vessels, such as those in your eyes and kidneys, are especially sensitive to high blood glucose levels. That is probably true, although all of these risk factors matter for both types of complications.

SIZING UP THE ENEMY

Let's take a minute to understand the dragons we are slaying, starting with cholesterol.

Your body uses cholesterol in the same way a factory might use petroleum. Cholesterol is a raw material, and your body makes many things from it. Believe it or not, cholesterol is used to make certain hormones, including testosterone and estrogen. It is also inserted into the thin cell membranes that surround each cell in your body, and it acts as a kind of glue to hold the membranes together. Without it, you would collapse into a gelatinous heap.

Just as refineries send trucks filled with petroleum to factories to be turned into everything from plastic to petroleum jelly, your liver sends

Is It My Genes?

Rick was 45 when he came to our office looking for help. He was not terribly optimistic that a diet change could really help him. His father had had diabetes and heart disease, and his own cholesterol had been high for years. Previous diets had let him down. A few years earlier, his doctor had suggested limiting red meat and eating more fish and chicken, but the change had had no perceptible effect. "I must have a genetic problem," he said.

It may well be that genes played a big role in his problem, I told him. But we would not know that until we made a more serious effort to change his eating habits—one that went beyond what he had tried before.

I explained to him what you are reading in this chapter. He decided to give it a try. (His story continues on page 171.)

particles containing cholesterol into your bloodstream for your cells to use.

Imagine what would happen if a refinery flooded the roads with tankers, sending out far more supply than was needed. Day after day, more and more oil trucks would clog up the roadways. Some might have accidents, spilling cargo and creating havoc.

Cholesterol presents the same problem. When too many particles of cholesterol pass through your bloodstream, they create a different kind of congestion.

The circulating particles can easily become damaged. When they do, they spark the formation of raised bumps called plaques, which are very much like small scars on your artery walls.

Now, this is dangerous, because plaques are fragile. They can crack or rupture, and when that happens, the blood around the plaque starts to clot. The growing clot can fill the artery like a cork and stop blood-flow. If that happens in an artery that carries blood to the heart, a portion of heart muscle will die. That's a heart attack, which doctors call a myocardial infarction.

The solution to the problem is to reduce the number of cholesterol particles circulating in the bloodstream. Luckily, we know how to do that. Although previous diets had only a modest ability to lower cholesterol, the diet changes described within the pages of this book are dramatically effective.

REVERSING HEART DISEASE

The most famous program using diet and lifestyle changes to tackle cholesterol and reverse heart disease was developed by Dean Ornish, MD, at the Preventive Medicine Research Institute in Sausalito, California.

Dr. Ornish is a Harvard-trained physician who made medical history in 1990 by showing that a combination of diet and other lifestyle changes could actually reverse artery blockages. His findings were published in the *Journal of the American Medical Association*, *Lancet*, and other prestigious journals.

In his landmark study, Dr. Ornish recruited heart patients from hospitals in the San Francisco area and divided them into two groups. Participants in one group—the control group—were asked to follow their regular doctors' advice about diet and other treatments. Generally speaking, that meant a diet favoring chicken and fish rather than red meat, cutting back on fat, and using medications as needed.

The other group—the experimental group—was given a very different regimen. They did not use cholesterol-lowering drugs at all. Instead, they began a very special diet. First, because cholesterol is found in animal products (meat, dairy products, and eggs), Dr. Ornish chose a vegetarian diet for the study. Remember, grains, beans, vegetables, fruits—in fact, all plant-derived foods—are essentially cholesterol-free.

These foods are also free of animal fat, which is even more important. Just to clarify, cholesterol and fat are two different things. Cholesterol is a microscopic ingredient in cell membranes, as described above, and is present in all animal cells.

Fat is different. It is the white strip in a cut of roast beef, the yellow layer under chicken skin, and the greasy residue left on your fingers if you touch a salmon fillet. You can easily see and feel animal fat. When you eat it, your body makes cholesterol.

I learned about animal fat as a child growing up in North Dakota. Some mornings, my mother cooked bacon for my four siblings and me. When it was done, she put the hot strips on paper towels to drain. She then carefully picked up the frying pan and poured the hot grease into a jar to save it. Now, she did not store the jar of bacon grease in the refrigerator; she simply put it in the cupboard. She knew that as it cooled, it would turn into a waxy solid. The next day, she spooned some of the bacon grease into a pan and fried eggs in it. With that sort of diet, it is perhaps remarkable that any of her children lived to adulthood, but that is the way we ate until we learned better.

The fact that bacon grease is solid at room temperature is a sign that it is loaded with *saturated* fat, which you can think of as "bad" fat, because it raises your cholesterol level.*

All fats are mixtures. Beef fat, for example, is about half saturated fat, with the rest being a mixture of various unsaturated fats. Chicken fat is about 30 percent saturated fat. Fish vary from about 15 to 30 percent saturated fat. Vegetable oils are much lower in saturated fat, except for the tropical oils: Coconut, palm, and palm kernel oil are all high in saturated fat.

Some food companies alter vegetable oils through a process called hydrogenation, which makes them similar to saturated fats. The resulting fats, called trans fats or partially hydrogenated fats, are solid and have a long shelf life. Unfortunately, their effect on your cholesterol level is similar to that of butter or lard. They are sometimes used in restaurant fryers and in snack foods. When you see the words *partially hydrogenated vegetable oil* on a food label, it's a good idea to move along to a healthier choice.

You can see why Dr. Ornish decided to use a vegetarian diet in a program of healthy lifestyle changes. Plant foods have essentially no cholesterol and no animal fat. He also kept vegetable oils to a minimum.

The results were remarkable. Among the vegetarians, chest pain rapidly melted away. The average person's LDL ("bad") cholesterol fell by about 40 percent. After a year, each participant had an angiogram— a special x-ray that shows blockages in the arteries of the heart—and Dr. Ornish compared the results with those of the same kind of test

---

* If you are wondering where the term *saturated fat* came from, it's actually very logical. If you could look at a fat molecule under a powerful microscope, it would look like a long chain of carbon atoms, with perhaps 18 or 20 atoms joined in a line. Attached to the carbon chain are hydrogen atoms. If the chain is completely covered (i.e., saturated) with hydrogen atoms, the fat becomes a waxy solid and is called a saturated fat. If, however, hydrogen atoms are absent at several spots on the fat chain, the fat is called polyunsaturated. Polyunsaturated oils are liquids. And if just one spot on the carbon chain has no hydrogen atoms attached, the fat is called monounsaturated. Olive and canola oils are rich in this sort of fat. They are unusual in that they are liquid at room temperature but solid in the refrigerator. Saturated fat is the kind that pushes your cholesterol upward.

done at the beginning of the study. The results were amazing: The blockages in the coronary arteries—the arteries that nourish the heart muscle itself—were actually starting to shrink. The arteries were opening again. The effect was so pronounced that the difference could be clearly seen on the angiograms of 82 percent of patients after the first year—all with no heart bypasses, no angioplasties, and not even cholesterol-lowering drugs.

WAKE UP AND SMELL THE CHOLESTEROL

By now you are probably yawning, saying you already know that cholesterol and saturated fat are bad and that we're supposed to cut down on them. "Been there, done that," you say.

Well, that is exactly the problem. For years, health authorities have suggested that people "cut down" on foods containing cholesterol and animal fat. Many people have chosen "leaner" cuts of beef and favored chicken and fish, but they have gotten very little in the way of results. Most people find that despite these diet changes, their cholesterol levels barely budge at all, and many have decided that diet changes are a waste of time. They conclude that their problems are genetic and give up on their diets.

It turns out that a switch from red meat to white meat is just not good enough. And here's why: All meats—even "lean" meats—contain cholesterol, ranging from about 10 milligrams in every ounce of tuna to about 50 milligrams per ounce of shrimp. Chicken and beef are in between, with about 25 milligrams per ounce. And yes, cholesterol in foods does pass into your bloodstream. Despite the egg industry's efforts to convince scientists and the public that "cholesterol in foods does not affect how much cholesterol is in your blood," the fact is that cholesterol in foods does indeed raise blood cholesterol. Red meat, poultry, and fish—even the "leaner" cuts—also contain a significant amount of fat. And saturated fat causes your body to make cholesterol.

In contrast, of course, there is no cholesterol or animal fat in any food from plants. That goes for every fruit and vegetable; every bean;

every grain; every variety of rice, pasta, and potato; and everything made from them.

Thus, if you were to try to lower your cholesterol by simply switching from beef to chicken and fish, you would have one arm tied behind your back. As shown in clinical tests, the cholesterol-lowering effect of a switch from red meat to white meat is minimal—only about half the effect of a plant-based diet. Most people who follow such diets have no measurable improvement within their arteries, either—on average, their artery blockages continue to get worse as time goes by.

WHY DIDN'T ANYONE TELL ME?

When Dr. Ornish's findings were published, most medical authorities were willing to believe his program was a very healthful regimen. But many felt the program was so austere that few people could actually follow it. I have studied that issue in some detail, however, and have come to a completely different conclusion. The diet is not terribly austere. In fact, it stacks up well against any other diet a doctor might prescribe. Let me describe my own experience.

When I was growing up in cattle country, my family ate pretty much the same things every day: roast beef, baked potatoes, and corn—except for special occasions, when we ate roast beef, baked potatoes, and peas.

In medical school, I decided to change my diet. At first, I tried pasta, making a sauce from fresh tomatoes, basil, and spices. Then I discovered that just below the beef, poultry, and fish choices, Chinese restaurant menus feature many delicious vegetable dishes, as do Mexican restaurants. Japanese restaurants serve delicious miso soup, salads, and vegetable sushi. Middle Eastern cuisine is simple but delicious, with hummus, falafel, couscous, and other delights. Thai, Indian, Ethiopian—all these cuisines offer endless vegetarian choices. Compared to those elegant meals, my North Dakota roast beef, baked potato, and corn no longer seemed like the pinnacle of the culinary art. To me, a plant-based diet was a world of new tastes and was anything but austere.

When I first learned about the work of Dr. Ornish in the late 1980s, I was working at the psychiatry clinic at George Washington University. I telephoned him and suggested that we study the acceptability of his diet. I flew to San Francisco and interviewed each of the participants in his heart study.[1] I asked how well they liked the foods they ate, how much effort was required to prepare them, what their family members thought, and what they planned to do in the future.

I found that the vegetarian group did grumble a bit at first. They had to learn about some new foods and master some new cooking tricks. On average, it took about 4 weeks before the diet really became second nature to them. But they adapted well, partly because they saw such dramatic results. Their cholesterol levels plummeted, their chest pain disappeared, and their heart disease reversed. The average participant lost, believe it or not, 22 pounds during the first year.[2, 3] They came to love the foods they ate.

I vividly remember one participant's reaction. He was angry— angry that previous doctors were eager to prescribe potentially dangerous drugs and even operate on him, charging him enormous amounts of money, and did not bother to even mention the power of diet changes. Overall, the participants not only found their diets acceptable, they felt it would be wrong for doctors not to give patients this kind of choice.

Now, it did not surprise me that the vegetarian diet took a little getting used to, or that the patients soon came to love it. What surprised me was the reaction of the control group—the group that was not asked to adopt the vegetarian diet. *They* grumbled, too. Some said their diet was nothing but chicken and fish, chicken and fish, chicken and fish, night after night. All the pleasures of life were gone, some said. *And they had nothing to show for it.* Many were still dealing with chest pain, trying to control their cholesterol levels with medication, and fighting a losing battle.

Having repeatedly studied how people react to different diets, I am convinced that a vegan diet is actually easier to follow than most other diets. This is partly because of its simplicity. Like quitting smoking or freeing yourself from any other habit, setting aside unhealthy foods is easier than teasing yourself with small amounts of them day after day. And the diet's benefits are usually so rewarding that you want to stick with it.

A few years later, I reviewed every published research study in which heart patients were asked to change their diet, with researchers tracking their success or failure.[4] At the time, the prevailing wisdom was that doctors should not push their patients too hard to make diet changes because the patients were likely to just throw up their hands and give up. But I found just the opposite. In controlled studies, when researchers asked patients to make small diet changes, they in fact achieved only small changes. When researchers encouraged their study participants to make bigger diet changes, most participants actually did make them, and they got better results. You can do it, too. Your heart deserves the very best.

AIMING TO BE HEART ATTACK–PROOF

Let's leave Dr. Ornish's California research center and take a short trip to Ohio to meet Anthony Yen. He grew up in China, where his family members routinely lived to a ripe old age. For them, heart disease, weight problems, diabetes, cancer, and high blood pressure were virtually unheard of. They dined on rice, noodles, and vegetable dishes of various kinds and used meat as no more than a flavoring, the way some might use bits of onion, garlic, or pine nuts.

In 1949, as a young man, Anthony moved to the United States and slowly gave up his traditional Chinese diet in favor of an American one. As the years went by, he gradually gained weight, like many of his American friends, and he started to develop heart problems, which steadily worsened. Ultimately, he needed surgery—a quintuple heart bypass.

Then he was lucky enough to join a program for heart patients run by a surgeon at the Cleveland Clinic. Caldwell Esselstyn Jr., MD, aimed to get cholesterol levels so low that heart disease would stop in its tracks. He prescribed a vegetarian diet without dairy products or added oils. He showed patients how to cook and even occasionally hosted group dinners that featured home-cooked foods. He added medications only if a patient's cholesterol level did not fall below 150 mg/dl with diet alone.

The program worked. Dr. Esselstyn's patients became practically bulletproof. Although they were in bad shape when they arrived, no one who adhered to the program had any sort of recurring heart problem.[5] Anthony's cholesterol level improved dramatically. He lost weight and felt better than he had in years.

In the ensuing years, Dr. Esselstyn called American cardiologists together for the Summit on Cholesterol and Coronary Disease. He put forward his belief that physicians need to promote healthier diets. If doctors continue to prescribe only modestly effective diets, he said, their patients will be stuck with endless prescriptions, operating rooms will remain busy with angioplasties and coronary bypass surgeries, and medical costs will continue to soar.

Dr. Esselstyn was right, as Anthony Yen, his other patients, and a growing number of physicians can attest.

SPECIAL-EFFECT FOODS

By now, you know which foods to avoid. By skipping animal products and added oils, you will sidestep cholesterol and the fat that can drive cholesterol levels up. Of course, you want to avoid these foods anyway in order to improve diabetes.

There are foods you might want to *add* to your diet, though, because they can actually lower your cholesterol or protect against the damage that cholesterol can cause.

- **Oats, beans, and barley** contain soluble fiber that reduces cholesterol levels. You have no doubt heard that oatmeal and other oat cereals have this effect, and they have become popular for exactly that reason. But do not forget the cholesterol-lowering power of the humble bean, which also contains soluble fiber. Eating a serving of beans every day cuts cholesterol levels significantly. Soluble fiber is also found in many vegetables and fruits.

- **Soy products** have a special cholesterol-lowering effect. Aside from the fact that they have no cholesterol or animal fat, there is something about soy protein that brings down cholesterol a bit further. If your burger is made of soybeans instead of beef, you will not only skip beef's cholesterol and fat, you will also get an extra cholesterol-lowering benefit.[6]

- **Certain nuts, such as almonds and walnuts,** lower cholesterol, too. Yes, they are as high in fat as other nuts, but somehow they have an ability to reduce cholesterol levels that has not been fully explained. In studies, eating 3 ounces a day for 4 weeks has shown a measurable effect.[7] I do not recommend that you make nuts a regular part of your diet, however. Despite their cholesterol-lowering effect, they are so fatty that they will make weight loss difficult and may interfere with your efforts to improve insulin sensitivity.

- **Some margarines** incorporate natural plant stanols or sterols that work almost like drugs, blocking the absorption of cholesterol from the small intestine. Benecol Light spread, for example, contains plant stanols derived from pine trees mixed into a spread made with canola and soybean oils (see benecol.com). You can use it in baking and frying if you like. It is not a low-calorie or low-fat spread, though; 1 tablespoon has about 50 calories. Like nuts, margarines can interfere with your weight-loss efforts.

- **Fruits and vegetables** are not only cholesterol free and very low in fat; their beta-carotene, vitamin C, and vitamin E can actually reduce the damaging effects of cholesterol in your blood. Here's why.

    As cholesterol particles glide along in your bloodstream, those that enter artery walls and cause plaque buildup are the ones that have become slightly damaged, or oxidized. Beta-carotene, vitamin C, and vitamin E actually *protect* the cholesterol particles from damage so they go on their merry way without harming you.

    You will find huge amounts of beta-carotene in orange vegetables, such as carrots, sweet potatoes, and pumpkins, but there is also plenty in green leafy vegetables. Vitamin C is in citrus fruits, of course, but also in many other fruits and vegetables. And whole grains, vegetables, and beans are healthful sources of vitamin E.

At the University of Toronto, Dr. David Jenkins took this approach to its ultimate conclusion. He reasoned that if a vegan diet (that is, one with no meat, dairy products, or eggs) lowers cholesterol levels; if soluble fiber, such as that in oat bran, lowers cholesterol; if certain nuts lower cholesterol; if soy products lower cholesterol; and if plant sterols lower cholesterol, then *what would happen if he prescribed them all at the same time?*

He devised what he called a Portfolio Diet, which included all of these elements, and found that the combination led to a 29.6 percent drop in LDL cholesterol *in just 4 weeks*, which was similar to the effect of cholesterol-lowering drugs.[8]

CONTROLLING CHOLESTEROL STEP BY STEP

Let's summarize what research tells us about the ideal cholesterol-lowering diet. Here are the keys.

1. Skip animal products. You will want to avoid meat (that means no red meat, no chicken, and no fish), dairy products, and eggs. Avoid them entirely, and you will eliminate all the animal fat and cholesterol from your diet. You already know this is important for diabetes, and it is just as important for your heart.

2. Keep vegetable oils to a minimum. To trim the oil from your diet, skip the oily dressings, fried foods, and foods prepared with extra oil. Read the labels on packaged foods. If you spot animal products or partially hydrogenated oils in the ingredient list, you will want to avoid that food. And if there are more than 2 to 3 grams of fat in a serving, skip it.

3. Add special-effect foods. The best of these are oats, beans, and soy products. They are filling but modest in calories, and they really do bring your cholesterol down. It is easy to add special-effect foods to your routine.

Oats: Start your day with a bowl of old-fashioned oatmeal. Top it with cinnamon if you like, but skip the milk and sugar or use soy milk.

Beans: Like oats, beans are high in soluble fiber, which lowers cholesterol. Baked beans, black beans with salsa, pinto beans wrapped in a tortilla—all are loaded with soluble fiber, protein, and all-around

Jumping Into Oatmeal

Rick, whom you met earlier, did very well with his diet changes despite his initial reservations. He learned how to make a quick and hearty vegetable soup from a dried soup mix to which he added tomatoes, cucumbers, sweet potatoes, and whatever other vegetables he had on hand. He often cooked pasta and usually used marinara sauce from a jar for convenience. He also included plenty of salads and cooked vegetables. Eating out was a challenge for him until he discovered that international (Italian, Chinese, Japanese, Mexican, Thai, etc.) restaurants had plenty of options. Speaking up helped, too—most restaurants gladly made him a vegetable plate when he asked for it. He figured out which fast-food restaurants had veggie burgers or salad bars and where he could get a respectable bean burrito.

He took a shine to what he called fake meats—bologna, ham, and other deli slices made of soy protein—which he used in sandwiches with sliced tomato, lettuce, and Dijon mustard. Sometimes he had a simple meal of beans and rice or a packaged rice dish (curried rice, rice pilaf, etc.). He also became quite fond of couscous. For breakfast, he jumped into oatmeal, figuratively speaking, and kept bananas and other fruits on hand both at home and at work.

While he found the diet surprisingly easy, he ran into a stumbling block at the beginning. He served himself modest portions and resisted going back for seconds. As a result, he often felt hungry. The fix: He simply ate more. On another occasion, he took my advice to eat beans a bit too far and had an episode of gastric distress. He cut back on his bean serving sizes for a bit and was fine.

His wife joined him in adopting a vegan diet. In the process, she lost a substantial amount of weight and had more energy than she had had in years.

By the time Rick came in for his follow-up blood test, he had totally adapted to the diet, and he was thrilled with the results. In 3 months, his cholesterol had dropped from 210 to 145, with an LDL of well below 100. And this was the same man who had started out saying what he really needed was different genes. "You know, this isn't a diet," he said. "This is a way of living, and it just feels right to me. I'm never going back to the way I used to eat. This is it."

good nutrition. The humble bean has even become quite chic, with some growers specializing in beautifully colorful heirloom varieties.

Soy: It is easy to bring soy milk into your routine. You will also want to learn about the many other forms of soy: low-fat tofu, tempeh, and many others. Some people are a bit tentative about tofu until they taste it properly prepared, then they come to love it. For all soy products, read the labels and choose those lowest in fat.

With these changes, most people can expect to see major results. Diets that eliminate cholesterol and animal fat (vegan diets), keep oils low, and use special-effect foods typically achieve a big reduction in "bad" cholesterol.

4. If you are overweight, follow the weight-loss guidelines described in Chapter 6. Each pound you lose cuts your total cholesterol slightly.[9] The effect is gradual but important.

5. Exercise. When your doctor gives you the green light to exercise, you will find it enormously helpful. Exercise will not lower your total cholesterol, but it will increase HDL cholesterol, and that may improve your overall health profile. Regular exercise (taking a brisk 30-minute walk five times a week or a 1-hour walk three times a week) also helps keep your blood pressure under control. Work with your doctor to set exercise goals based on your current health (see Chapter 11).

SIZING UP YOUR PROGRESS

It is easy to see if the program is working. Follow it carefully, and after about 8 weeks, ask your doctor to check your cholesterol level. If you have not quite reached the goals you set for yourself, take a close look at what you have been eating. How well have you followed the program? If you really did follow it carefully and your cholesterol failed to budge, you are probably one of those uncommon individuals whose genes really are driving up their cholesterol levels.

If diet alone proves insufficient, follow your doctor's advice, which may include cholesterol-lowering medications. Some doctors believe that medications have value even when cholesterol levels are normal. Research is under way to test this possibility.

WHAT ABOUT "GOOD" CHOLESTEROL?

The cholesterol in high-density lipoprotein (HDL) particles is called "good" cholesterol for only one reason: It is on the way out of your body. HDL particles scour your artery walls, picking up cholesterol and eliminating it, like tiny sanitation trucks carrying away garbage.

When people begin low-fat vegan diets, their HDL levels sometimes fall slightly. But that is not a reason to worry—your LDL ("bad") cholesterol level is likely to fall much more. In fact, some people say that, since you have less "garbage" in your bloodstream (that is, less LDL cholesterol), you don't need so many "garbage trucks" (that is, HDL cholesterol) to haul it away.

REDUCING TRIGLYCERIDES

Triglycerides is a technical term for fat in the bloodstream.* Lowering triglycerides is a good idea, as it will reduce your risk of heart problems. It is usually easy to do. A low-fat plant-based diet is a good start. But take one additional step: avoid sugar, white bread products, and other high-GI foods, as discussed in Chapter 4. These foods seem to raise triglycerides, while low-GI foods that are rich in fiber seem to lower them. You will probably see a big drop in your triglycerides.

ONE SOLUTION TO MANY PROBLEMS

If you have been following along, you have probably come to this happy conclusion on your own: You do not need one diet for diabetes, another for cholesterol control, and a third one for weight loss. A diet that skips animal products, keeps vegetable oils low, and favors high-fiber, low-GI foods tackles all these problems at the same time.

Just as a drop in cholesterol is good for your heart, a drop in A1C is, too. People who keep their glucose under good control have fewer heart problems as the years go by.

The same diet changes also help control your blood pressure, partly because they can cause you to lose weight, and as your weight falls, so

---

*The word *triglyceride* is derived from the fact that when your body transports fat molecules from one place to another, it generally attaches three fat molecules to a glycerine molecule (hence, tri-glyceride) before sending them into the watery environment of the bloodstream.

does your blood pressure. But the effect of vegetarian diets on blood pressure goes beyond their effect on weight. Plant-based diets are rich in potassium, which seems to reduce blood pressure. The absence of animal fat also reduces blood viscosity (that is, blood is less "thick"— less like grease and more like water) so it flows more easily through the blood vessels.[10]

For many people, the effect of diet changes rivals or exceeds that of medications. If, for whatever reason, your cholesterol, blood pressure, or blood sugar does not come under good control despite your best efforts, your doctor will rightly talk with you about medications to take up where diet leaves off.

CHAPTER 13

Healthy Nerves, Eyes, and Kidneys

Selwyn was 58 years old when he heard we were looking for volunteers for a research study. Originally from Trinidad, he had been diagnosed with diabetes almost 20 years earlier. The disease had taken a toll on his eyes, and he was being treated for glaucoma.

He also had terrible nerve pain. In the 18 months before the study began, the pain in his feet had gotten worse and worse. "It was excruciating," he said. "It hurt from the calves down, especially on the left side. And it worsened as the day wore on. By the time I got home from work, I just had to put my feet up. At night, the bottoms of my feet hurt terribly, with burning and tingling."

He had had several medical tests to search for a treatable cause, but his doctors were left with only diabetes to blame for his misery. Despite the fact that he used insulin twice a day, his diabetes was not under good control.

He began doing stretching exercises, which seemed to ease the pain somewhat. When our study began, he started a low-fat, vegan diet. It suited his tastes and had a remarkable effect on his diabetes. At the beginning of the study, his A1C was 9.1 percent, but his blood sugar began to fall soon after he made the switch to our eating plan. Within a month, he began to have episodes of low blood sugar, so his insulin doses were reduced. Despite the fact that he was taking less medication, his A1C at the 3-month point was down to 7.7. That was a big improvement, although he was not yet where he needed to be.

However, he kept improving. And about 6 months into the study, something remarkable happened. "I noticed a drastic change. I had been in total pain, but the symptoms started going away," he said. As time went on, things got better and better. The pain became barely perceptible, and eventually—to his amazement—it disappeared altogether. "I'm totally normal," he said. "I have no pain at all anymore."

If a medication could deliver the result he achieved, it would be a very popular one indeed. "The difference has been like night and day for me," he said.

A healthful diet does much more than keep your blood sugar down; it helps protect your whole body. If diabetes rages out of control, it can not only damage your heart, it can also attack your nerves, your eyes, and your kidneys. The diet you are now beginning will help you avoid these problems. In this chapter, we will look at how to keep all your body parts in good working order.

HEALTHY NERVES

People with diabetes are at risk of nerve damage, which can take two forms.

Peripheral neuropathy, sometimes called sensorimotor neuropathy, is damage to the nerves that allow you to feel things or to move your muscles. It leads to tingling, pain, numbness, or weakness in your feet or hands. It pays to take these signs seriously because although it can get better, it can also get a lot worse if you are not careful.

Reduced sensation in your feet can leave you vulnerable to injuries that you cannot feel. It is easy to overlook a small cut or scrape when you do not feel it. Injuries can also be slow to heal, which can set you up for a festering infection. Diabetes is a common cause of amputation, something that should never happen with good care.

Autonomic neuropathy is abnormalities in the nerves that control your internal functions. It can lead to digestive problems, such as nausea, vomiting, constipation, or diarrhea. It can also cause problems with bladder control or sexual function. Other symptoms include dizziness, faintness, increased or decreased sweating, visual difficulties (e.g., problems adjusting to light and dark conditions), and lack of awareness of the warning signs of low blood sugar.

SEE YOUR DOCTOR

Sometimes nerve symptoms have nothing to do with diabetes. If you have unexplained numbness, pain, tingling, or other nerve symptoms, it is important to see your doctor to check for conditions that can be treated. For example, if you are low in vitamin B_{12}, you can have nerve pain that is indistinguishable from the nerve symptoms of diabetes and can end up being permanent. Your doctor will check your vitamin B_{12} blood level and will help you get back on track, if that is the issue. Nerves are also affected by thyroid conditions, medications, infections, compression, and other factors. So it's important to have a good evaluation.

If the diagnosis is diabetic neuropathy, the key to preventing and treating it is to get your diabetes—particularly your blood glucose level—under control, starting with diet and exercise. If neuropathy has affected you, you will want to reread Chapter 4 and follow the diet guidelines to the letter, aiming for the best possible glucose control under the guidance of your doctor. There are medications that can help slightly, but for most people, diet and exercise are far more powerful.

At California's Weimar Institute of Health and Education, Milton Crane, MD, asked 21 diabetes patients with peripheral neuropathy to do two things: begin a low-fat, vegan diet and take a daily 30-minute walk. The effects were rapid and very strong: Within 2 weeks, leg pains stopped completely in 17 of the participants, and the remaining 4 had partial relief.[1]

My own research team carried this research a step further. We invited people with neuropathy to see what a diet change alone could do for them—without exercise. Not that exercise is bad. Just the opposite, it's very healthful, but we wanted to isolate the effect of diet for scientific reasons, to see how powerful foods could be. Using the diet steps that are now familiar to you (avoiding animal products, minimizing the use of oils, and favoring low-Glycemic-Index foods), we found that, for many patients pain improved or simply went away, and objective tests of nerve function improved, too.[2]

Supplements for Treating Neuropathy

Researchers have tested the effects of the following supplements. The verdicts are not yet in on them as treatments for nerve damage, so I'm listing them here not as a recommendation but simply to make you aware of them.

Alpha-lipoic acid appears to improve neuropathy symptoms.[3] In research studies, a dose of 600 milligrams taken once daily was effective.

Gamma-linolenic acid is an omega-6 fatty acid commonly sold in health food stores. At doses of 480 milligrams per day, it appears to reduce neuropathy symptoms.[4]

Carnitine, in doses of 1,000 milligrams daily, appears to improve nerve condition and reduce pain in patients with diabetic neuropathy.[5]

If You Have Nerve Damage

If the nerves of your feet have been damaged, it is important that you get regular checkups and protect your feet. If you have lost some feeling, check your feet daily for any sign of injury or infection, such as redness or swelling, and have it treated right away. Avoid walking barefoot. If you have lost some feeling in your feet, you may not know if you step on something that breaks the skin. Be sure your shoes fit properly to avoid blisters, and break in new shoes slowly. Keep your nails in good shape, and do not trim them shorter than the ends of your toes. If your vision is poor or you have difficulty safely trimming your nails, have a podiatrist examine your feet and trim your nails.

Needless to say, you will want to focus on more than just caring for your feet. Fight back against neuropathy with a healthy diet—vegan, low-fat, and low-GI.

HEALTHY EYES

Your eyes are delicate cameras that capture the world around you, transmitting its details to your brain to perceive and remember. In the same way that a camera is fragile, several parts of the eye are susceptible to damage. This is true for anyone, but especially for people with diabetes. Protecting your eyes means keeping your blood glucose, blood pressure, and cholesterol under control.

Three parts of the eye are particularly vulnerable. First, pressure can build up in the front part of the eye—called the anterior chamber—and eventually damage the retina and optic nerve. This is glaucoma. Second, a cataract can compromise the lens's clarity. Third, blood vessels in the retina can become damaged. Let's look at what we can do to prevent this three-pronged assault.

Glaucoma

There are several different types of glaucoma. Typically, increasing pressure within the eye pinches the tiny blood vessels in the retina, damaging it and the optic nerve. High blood pressure and high glucose levels both increase your risk of developing glaucoma. Your best defense is to get both under control, using the information in this chapter and the rest of this book. If glaucoma is caught early, treatment (with prescription eye drops) is highly effective.

Glaucoma can begin with no symptoms at all, so it is important to have eye examinations by an ophthalmologist at least once a year.

Cataracts

If the lens of the eye loses its clarity, becoming more like waxed paper than like a clear pane of glass, a doctor diagnoses a cataract. You may experience blurred or double vision, difficulty with distance vision, a halo effect around lights, or excessive glare in bright sunlight or while driving at night.

While cataract surgery has advanced dramatically in recent years, the ideal situation is to keep your original equipment in good working order. Luckily, there are several things you can do to help prevent cataracts.

First, it is important to avoid tobacco and to protect your eyes from harsh sunlight.

Second, it pays to follow the same diet steps that apply to controlling diabetes in general, as described in Chapter 4. That means avoiding animal products, keeping oils to a minimum, and favoring low-GI foods. There is evidence that these steps reduce your risk. Specifically, people who avoid fatty foods tend to have less cataract risk.[6]

The same appears to be true for people who avoid dairy products. Generally speaking, people who steer clear of dairy products appear to have significantly less risk of developing cataracts.[7] The culprit here appears to be lactose, or milk sugar, rather than milk fat.

During the digestive process, lactose releases a simple sugar called galactose, which can enter the lens. Infants who lack the enzymes necessary to break down galactose develop cataracts within the first year of life. The relationship between dairy products and cataracts is still being studied, but this is one more good reason to avoid them.

Certain foods help protect the eyes. Particularly valuable are green leafy vegetables such as broccoli, spinach, kale, collards, and mustard greens. They are rich sources of certain antioxidants, called lutein and zeaxanthin, which protect both the lens and the retina.[8] Foods rich in vitamins C and E may help, too.[9] You will find plenty of vitamin C in oranges, bell peppers, cantaloupe, strawberries, and kiwifruit. It also shows up in places you may not expect: cruciferous vegetables—broccoli, Brussels sprouts, cauliflower, and kale—as well as tomatoes and sweet potatoes. Healthy sources of vitamin E include cooked

The Eye

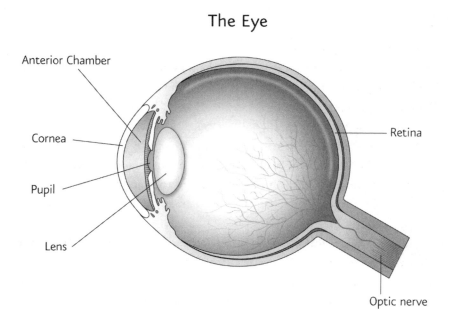

Anterior Chamber

Cornea

Pupil

Lens

Retina

Optic nerve

spinach, soy milk, mangoes, and wheat germ. Most nuts and seeds are particularly rich in vitamin E, but be careful, as they are fatty and loaded with calories. A small handful has about 5 milligrams of vitamin E.

Finally, people who avoid alcohol have about 10 percent less cataract risk than other people. Even very modest consumption, about two drinks per week, is linked to increased risk.[10]

Retinopathy

The retina, located at the back of your eye, is like camera film. Millions of tiny nerves in the retina pick up images and send them to the brain. Also like film, your retinas are fragile. They can be damaged by high blood sugar, blood pressure, or cholesterol, leading to a condition called retinopathy, meaning damage to the retina. The condition occurs in two main forms.

Nonproliferative retinopathy occurs when capillaries balloon out and leak substances into the retina, leading to the formation of fatty deposits. The condition is usually mild and needs no treatment, but it is essential that an ophthalmologist check your eyes regularly to be sure that it does not become more serious.

Proliferative retinopathy occurs when blood vessels are so damaged that they begin to close off. When that happens, new, abnormal vessels start to form in the retina. The new vessels are fragile and prone to bleeding, leading to scarring and sometimes even to retinal detachment. Ophthalmologists use laser treatments to treat the abnormal vessels.

Most people with diabetes eventually develop at least a mild degree of retinopathy. The good news is that there is a lot you can do to prevent serious problems. Good blood glucose control protects the eyes, and by now you know how to go about attaining that. Keeping blood pressure and cholesterol down helps, too. The diet steps above will go a long way toward helping you reach that goal. If diet alone is insufficient, your doctor will add medications as needed.

Retinopathy begins without symptoms, so it is essential to have your eyes checked regularly and to choose your foods as if your vision depended on it. It does.

HEALTHY KIDNEYS

Your kidneys are made up of millions of tiny filtration units. They purify your blood, sending waste products out into the urine and holding on to proteins and other normal blood components. But just as the retina's tiny blood vessels can be damaged, so can the tiny vessels in your kidneys. High blood pressure, high blood glucose, and high cholesterol assault them, leading to a condition doctors call nephropathy.

Left uncontrolled, kidney damage can progress to the point where your options boil down to dialysis or kidney transplant. Needless to say, you do not want anything like that to happen. Here are the diet steps you need to take.

First, follow the basic diet guidelines for diabetes as described in Chapter 4. The need is not just for avoiding fat and cholesterol and keeping your blood glucose and cholesterol down, although those are very important. Animal protein is part of the problem, too, so you want to avoid it. Since animal protein taxes the kidneys, getting your protein from plant sources helps protect them.[11]

This is an important point, so stick with me while I explain: Many people imagine that egg white, chicken breast, or haddock are healthful foods because they are high in protein—but that very fact is what makes them undesirable. The less animal protein you consume, the lower your risk of kidney problems. You are much safer getting your protein from plant sources—beans, vegetables, and grains, for example.

A low-fat, vegan diet is not only free of animal protein, cholesterol, and animal fat, it also helps bring down high blood pressure,[12] which is also important for protecting your kidneys.

It goes without saying that you should avoid tobacco. Among its many ill effects, smoking damages blood vessels.

If your blood pressure, glucose, or cholesterol remains high despite your best efforts, your doctor will prescribe medications to bring it under control. Some doctors prescribe medications even if your tests are in the normal range, as a means of protecting kidney tissues. This is done on an individualized basis.

In a recent study by our research team, we tracked the kidney health of our participants. They dutifully collected their urine twice over two 24-hour periods so we could measure their albumin losses (your doctor will probably use less arduous tests). They did this before beginning their assigned new diets and again after following them for 22 weeks.

During this time, a group following a "conventional" diet that involved limited calories and carbohydrates had a 21 percent average drop in albumin losses. That's a change in the right direction. However, a group following a low-fat vegan group had the advantage of consuming no animal protein, animal fat, or cholesterol, and its average albumin losses were reduced 56 percent, that is, they fell to less than half of their beginning values.

GETTING HEALTHY AND STAYING THAT WAY

If you have been gaining weight, needing more and more medications, or developing complications, my goal is to help you change course. We now know that it is possible to lose weight effectively and permanently, reduce or eliminate medications, reverse heart disease, and even improve the symptoms of neuropathy. If you thought you had to surrender to advancing symptoms, it's time to think again. You are now in the driver's seat.

CHAPTER 14

Information for Clinicians

Although this book is intended as a tool for people with diabetes, there are a few key points I would like to mention to physicians and other health care providers. As you will see, this program is both very effective and highly engaging. While health care providers are used to seeing their patients becoming frustrated with typical "diabetes diets" and requiring ever-higher medication dosages, both physicians and patients find this approach fresh and rewarding.

Health care providers play key roles for individuals on this program, just as they do with any diabetes treatment program. They educate and encourage their patients, guide them along the way, and monitor their progress.

In the research studies we have conducted, we have found that many patients treated with insulin or insulin secretogogues have hypoglycemic episodes as they improve their diets. As your patients embark on this new diet, you will need to prepare them for that possibility and be ready to reduce their medications as needed. It is also important that they understand that the hypoglycemia was caused by the medications, not by any defect in their physiology. More on this below.

THE ROLE OF THE HEALTH CARE PROVIDER

There are many ways physicians and other health care providers can help patients as they begin major dietary changes. First, of course, is encouragement. Many patients have seen their parents or grandparents end up with frightening diabetes complications, such as eye problems, loss of kidney function, or amputations, and many have already begun to experience neuropathy or other problems by the time they decide to take the disease seriously. They need to know that they can avoid these problems—as indeed they can—if they follow your advice, including maintaining a good diet.

It is helpful for them to know that this is not the same diabetes diet they may have already tried and that they will need to learn a few new tricks. They will discover new products, new restaurants, and perhaps new menu items at their old favorite restaurants. The most helpful physicians learn about these diet choices, too. If you have not yet tried a low-fat, vegan diet, I would strongly encourage you to do so. Apart from its health benefits, the experience will also prepare you to answer patients' questions and offer encouragement.

One way to help patients get started is to ask them to take a week to try out healthful vegan foods. The idea is not to give up anything. Rather, they are just trying out some healthful breakfasts, lunches, dinners, and snacks. In a few days, they will have found many good ideas (more on this in Chapter 5).

Then identify a limited period—say, 3 weeks—in which to give the diet a good try. For now, there is no need to commit to it forever, but during this short period, they would do well to follow it 100 percent so they can experience its full effect. Once they see how it works, they will want to continue.

Avoid the temptation to water down the diet. Clinicians who tell patients to follow a diet "most of the time" or to "just do the best you can" tacitly encourage them to deviate from it. We never do that when patients have alcohol or tobacco problems, because we know that it is easier to stick to a consistent program than to try to negotiate with these problem substances. The same is true of food; it is better to encourage patients to give it 100 percent, never setting a foot wrong.

Occasionally, some patients will slip back into their old diet habits. When that happens, they will almost instantly notice that they no longer manage their weight as well, and their blood glucose levels will start to climb again. They will also arrive at your office with a heavy burden of guilt. Many will speak of foods as "sinful," "decadent," etc. I suggest that you remain positive, avoid moralizing, and return the focus to biology, which is where it belongs. Patients who have returned fat to their diets may well be packing their cells with more intramyocellular lipid, which is likely to harm their insulin sensitivity. Encourage them to dust themselves off and get back on the wagon.

Some patients need to be encouraged to eat carbohydrate-rich foods. Because of the carbohydrate counting they have already learned, they may have come to see all carbohydrates as unhealthful. This feeling was aided and abetted by the never-ending low-carbohydrate diet craze. It is important to remind patients that countries whose populations have traditionally consumed high-carbohydrate diets—such as Asian countries, where rice and noodles are dietary staples and meat and dairy consumption is much less prevalent than in Western countries—have historically had very low diabetes rates.

You can also help patients ensure nutritional adequacy by asking them to take a daily B_{12} supplement. This is good advice for all patients.

HYPOGLYCEMIA

Patients who are taking insulin or insulin secretogogues are subject to hypoglycemia. When they improve their diets and begin to lose weight, hypoglycemic episodes are common. In my experience, most patients on insulin and about half of all patients on a sulfonylurea who begin a low-fat, vegan diet have hypoglycemic episodes, usually within the first several weeks.

Patients will be delighted to know that they have improved so much that their medications are now too strong, but they will also be concerned about what hypoglycemia means. It is important for them to understand that it was caused by their medication and that it does not indicate that there is anything wrong with them. It is also essential for them to know, right from the outset, what to do and whom to call when these episodes happen. Of course, the initial steps—checking their blood glucose and taking glucose tablets or food—are things they can do on their own. But it is important to provide specific instructions and to ask patients to carry your telephone number (or that of an office backup) with them and use it as necessary—even on weekends—so you can adjust their medications. You will find my instructions for patients on dealing with hypoglycemia beginning on page 102.

ADDITIONAL RESOURCES

Registered dietitians, as you know, are indispensable allies in your work with diabetes patients. Ideally, you will want to work with a dietitian who is a certified diabetes educator and a member of the Academy of Nutrition and Dietetics' Vegetarian Nutrition Dietetic Practice Group, which includes a large number of RDs skilled in the use of vegetarian diets.

The Physicians Committee for Responsible Medicine (PCRM) provides free, noncommercial nutrition information, including continuing medical education on its Web site, PCRM.org, as well as guidance on how to begin low-fat, vegan diets. It provides hundreds of recipes, shopping lists, and other user-friendly information. Please use it and encourage your patients to do so as well. They will especially like our 21-Day Vegan Kickstart, which offers 3 weeks of menus, recipes, and cooking videos in several languages, all for free.

If you would like to join in our work to promote healthful diets and tackle other issues in medicine and research, I hope you will consider joining PCRM. Members receive our quarterly magazine, *Good Medicine*, and can sign up to receive PCRM's Breaking Medical News, a free, noncommercial service that alerts you by e-mail when new studies are about to break.

Menus and Recipes

The following menus and recipes were developed and tested by Bryanna Clark Grogan, a veteran chef, recipe developer, and food writer. Originally from California, Bryanna now lives in British Columbia. Her many cookbooks cover an enormous range of foods and cooking styles, from quick and easy recipes to many kinds of ethnic cuisine.

Bryanna's recipes are full-bodied, savory dishes with a special "something." You will notice that their flavors go beyond the tastes and aromas of the individual ingredients. The blends of simple foods and well-chosen spices make each recipe special.

This recipe collection is intended for a wide range of tastes and temperaments and includes both simple and more adventurous offerings. When we have included an unusual ingredient, you can find more information in Appendix 2. Thanks to Gabrielle Turner-McGrievy, PhD, RD, and Jennifer Reilly, RD, who contributed additional recipes.

HOW TO STEAM-FRY

Some recipes call for steam-frying, a technique for sautéing or stir-frying without fat. Here is how to do it.

Place a heavy nonstick skillet or stir-fry pan over medium heat and add the ingredients to be cooked (e.g., chopped onions or other vegetables). Then add 1 to 2 tablespoons of liquid (water, low-sodium vegetable broth, or wine)—just enough to keep the food from sticking. Do not crowd the pan, or the vegetables will stew.

Increase the heat to high and cook until the liquid starts to evaporate, stirring with a wooden spatula or spoon until the vegetables are done to your liking.

You can brown onions perfectly by this method. As soon as the natural sugars in the onions start to brown on the bottom and edges of the pan, add a little more liquid and mix the browned portions with the remaining onions. Continue until the onions are soft and brown, being careful not to scorch them.

To steam-fry in a microwave, use a glass dish, such as a round 10-inch Pyrex baking dish or pie plate. Add the ingredients, including the 1 to 2 tablespoons of liquid, and cover with a glass lid or microwaveable plate. Microwave on high for 5 minutes or until the vegetables are soft, then add to the recipe. As almost everyone with a microwave knows, you can cook vegetables in it, but you cannot brown them or any other food. If you like a brown, crispy texture, stick with the stovetop method.

7 Days of Healthful Meals

DAY 1

Breakfast

Oatmeal cooked with apples

Soy milk

Lunch

Black-Eyed Pea and Sweet Potato Soup (page 214)

Toasted rye or sprouted-grain bread

Spinach salad with mandarin orange segments and *Creamy Poppy Seed Dressing* (page 210)

Snack

Fruit Smoothie (page 204)

Dinner

Lebanese-Style Lentils and Pasta (page 229)

Steamed broccoli

Orange-Applesauce Date Cake (page 248)

DAY 2

Breakfast

2 High-Protein Oat Waffles (page 202)

Sliced berries

Soy yogurt

Lunch

Spinach Hummus (page 206) and vegetables of choice wrapped in a sprouted-wheat tortilla

Orange Quinoa and Bulgur Tabbouleh (page 220)

Snack

Baked corn chips, salsa, and *Vegetarian "Refried" Beans* (page 205)

Dinner

Indonesian-Style Stir-Fried Pasta (page 234)

Thai-Style Coleslaw (page 223)

Fresh fruit

DAY 3

Breakfast

Tofu Scramblers (page 198)

Rye toast

Fruit salad

Lunch

Panini sandwich made with sprouted-grain bread, *Tofu Mayonnaise* (page 226), low-fat vegetarian deli slices, and arugula

Creamy Mushroom Bisque (page 212)

Snack

Apple slices dipped in *Lemon Crème* (page 245)

Dinner

Lemon and Artichoke Tagine (page 230)

Orange Couscous Pilaf (page 238)

Baby mixed greens salad with *Creamy Black Pepper Dressing* (page 210)

Berry Mousse (page 247)

DAY 4

Breakfast

Breakfast Barley with Fruit (page 197)

Soy milk

Lunch

Red Lentil and Sweet Potato Soup (page 215)

Italian Stuffed Griddle Dumplings (page 218)

Snack

Raw vegetables

Whole grain rye-crisp crackers

Spinach Dip (page 209)

Dinner

Eggplant Parmesan (page 236)

Green salad with *Balsamic Vinaigrette* (page 208)

Bulgur Wheat and Quinoa Pilaf (page 240)

Fresh fruit

DAY 5

Breakfast

Frozen fat-free hash browns baked in a nonstick waffle iron

Low-fat vegetarian sausage

Sliced oranges

Lunch

Black Bean Soft Tacos (page 216)

Cherry Tomato and Brown Rice Salad with Artichoke Hearts (page 222)

Snack

Orange-Applesauce Date Cake (page 248)

Nondairy milk

Dinner

Balkan-Style Slow-Cooker Stew (page 227)

Crusty rye bread

Brussels Sprouts with Lemon and Vegetarian Bacon (page 239)

Fresh fruit

DAY 6

Breakfast

Muesli Cereal (page 199)

Soy milk

Fresh fruit

Lunch

Sloppy Joes for Two (page 220) on sprouted-wheat hamburger buns

Green salad

Snack

Whole grain crackers

Cypriot Yellow Split Pea and Dill Spread (page 207)

Dinner

White Bean and Sweet Potato Stew (page 228)

Sprouted grain buns

Sautéed Portobello Mushroom Salad (page 225)

Cranberry–Orange–Pear Granola Crisp (page 244)

DAY 7

Breakfast

Wheatberry Pancakes (page 203) with apple-cider maple syrup

Fresh fruit

Lunch

Barley and Winter Squash Chowder (page 212)

Oatmeal Drop Scones (page 200)

Red Cabbage Slaw with Cranberries and Apples (page 224)

Snack

Pineapple Sherbet Pops (page 246)

Dinner

Vegetarian Mixed-Bean Chili Express (page 232)

Tender Barley Cornbread (page 201)

BLT Salad (page 226)

Chocolate-Dipped Strawberries (page 244)

Breakfasts

Breakfast Barley with Fruit

For delicious taste, lots of soluble fiber, and a wonderfully low gly-cemic index, try rolled barley (also called barley flakes) for your breakfast porridge. It takes a bit longer to cook than oatmeal unless you soak it the night before. Serve with your favorite nondairy milk and a touch of brown sugar or the sweetener of your choice.

⅓ cup rolled barley (barley flakes)
⅛ teaspoon salt
¾ cup water
1 tablespoon wheat bran
½ medium apple with peel, cored and chopped, or other
      chopped fruit
1½ teaspoons ground flaxseed

The night before: Combine the barley, salt, and water in a microwave-able bowl, cover, and refrigerate overnight. (Use a 1-quart or larger bowl—barley can really boil up!)

In the morning: Add the bran and apple or other fruit to the soaked barley. Cover the bowl with a microwaveable plate and microwave on high for 2 minutes. Finish cooking on medium for 4 minutes. Stir in the flaxseed.

To cook on the stovetop: Bring the soaked barley, bran, and apple or other fruit to a boil in a small nonstick saucepan over high heat, stir-ring. Reduce the heat to low, partially cover, and simmer for about 15 minutes, stirring occasionally. The mixture should have the con-sistency of cooked oatmeal. If it's too watery, continue cooking over low heat to desired consistency.

MAKES 1 SERVING

Per serving: 197 calories, 6 g protein, 8 g carbohydrates, 8 g sugar, 2 g total fat, 10% calories from fat, 0 mg cholesterol, 42 g fiber, 252 mg sodium

Tofu Scramblers

It takes about the same amount of time to make Tofu Scramblers as it does to make scrambled eggs when you use the handy homemade mix. Shake or stir the mix before measuring. Scramblers can be used in breakfast burritos or soft tacos made with sprouted wheat or corn tortillas, topped with salsa, or used in vegan huevos rancheros.

Scrambler Mix

    1   cup nutritional yeast flakes
    5   tablespoons + 1 teaspoon onion powder
    4   teaspoons curry powder
    4   teaspoons salt
    4   teaspoons ground turmeric
    4   teaspoons ground cumin

Scramblers

    1½ teaspoons Tofu Scrambler Mix
    4   ounces reduced-fat extra-firm silken tofu, crumbled
    2   tablespoons reduced-fat soy milk (optional)

For the mix: Blend the yeast flakes, onion powder, curry powder, salt, turmeric, and cumin in a dry blender or mini-processor. Store in a covered jar.

For the scramblers: Combine the scrambler mix and tofu well in a medium bowl. Add the soy milk, if desired. Cook the mixture in a heavy nonstick skillet until it reaches the desired consistency, stirring constantly with a plastic spatula.

To microwave, combine the ingredients in a microwaveable dish, cover, and cook on high (for 4 ounces, about 2 minutes; for 8 ounces, about 3½ minutes; for 12 ounces, about 5 minutes; and for 16 ounces, about 7½ minutes).

MAKES 1 SERVING

Per serving: 54 calories, 9 g protein, 3 g carbohydrates, 1 g sugar, 1 g total fat, 15% calories from fat, 0 mg cholesterol, 1 g fiber, 252 mg sodium

Variations

If you like, add chopped vegetarian bacon or ham; vegetarian bacon bits; or steam-fried chopped onions, scallions, mushrooms, bell peppers, or tomatoes. If cooking in the microwave, place the vegetables in the bottom of the dish, put the tofu (mixed with the scrambler mix) on top, and cook as usual, then stir together before serving.

Muesli Cereal

Bircher muesli was invented in Switzerland as a nutritious raw but digestible breakfast cereal. You can buy expensive commercial versions, but the original is low in fat, easy to make, and quick, as long as you remember to start the night before. Serve muesli with reduced-fat nondairy milk or soy yogurt; brown sugar, maple syrup or agave syrup to taste; and fresh fruit (such as berries), if desired.

1½ cups rolled oats or other rolled whole grain cereal
1½ cups water
2 tablespoons wheat bran
2 tablespoons currants, raisins, or other dried fruit
¼ teaspoon salt
2 medium apples with peel, grated
3 tablespoons lemon juice

The night before: Combine the oats and water in a bowl and refrigerate overnight.

Just before serving: Add the bran, currants or raisins, salt, apples, and lemon juice to the soaked oats.

Note: To make 1 serving, use 6 tablespoons oats; 6 tablespoons water; 1 teaspoon bran; 1 teaspoon dried fruit; a pinch of salt; ½ small apple, shredded; and 2¼ teaspoons lemon juice.

MAKES 4 SERVINGS

Per serving: 173 calories, 6 g protein, 36 g carbohydrates, 11 g sugar, 2 g total fat, 10% calories from fat, 0 mg cholesterol, 6 g fiber, 122 mg sodium

Oatmeal Drop Scones

Traditional Scottish *skon* recipes contained no fat at all. They were eaten immediately, warm and fresh, as these should be. Enjoy them with low-sugar jam.

    1 cup old-fashioned oats
 1¼ cups whole wheat pastry flour (not regular whole wheat flour)
    1 teaspoon sugar
  ½ teaspoon baking soda
  ½ teaspoon salt
 1¼ cups reduced-fat soy milk
    1 tablespoon lemon juice or vinegar
      Sugar or caraway seed

Preheat the oven to 400°F. Grind the oats to a fine meal in a dry blender. Pour into a medium bowl and add the flour, sugar, baking soda, and salt. Mix well.

Mix the soy milk and lemon juice or vinegar in a small bowl. Pour into the dry mixture and stir briefly with a fork. Drop by large spoonfuls onto 2 nonstick baking sheets (or baking sheets lined with parchment), making 12 mounds. Smooth the tops a bit with wet fingertips. Bake for about 15 minutes. Split with a fork while still hot.

For a bannock shape: Divide the dough in half. With wet hands, pat the dough pieces into 8" circles in two 9" nonstick cake pans (or cake pans lined with parchment cut to fit). Score each circle into 6 wedges and bake for 15 to 20 minutes.

Sprinkle with the sugar or caraway seed.

MAKES 12 SERVINGS

Per serving: 77 calories, 3 g protein, 15 g carbohydrates, 1 g sugar, 1 g total fat, 9% calories from fat, 0 mg cholesterol, 2 g fiber, 144 mg sodium

Variations

Currant Scones: Add ¼ to ½ cup dried currants. You can also add ¾ cup grated apple.
Herb Scones: Add ½ cup loosely packed chopped fresh herbs of your choice.

Herb Bannock: This resembles a focaccia, is quick to make, and is a great snack. Add ½ cup fresh herbs to the oatmeal scone dough. Divide the dough in half and follow the instructions for making the bannock shape. Make indentations all over the dough with your fingertips. Spray the tops lightly with water from a pump sprayer and sprinkle with coarse salt or soy Parmesan, or top with steam-fried or grilled chopped mushrooms, garlic, bell peppers, and/or onions. Serve with balsamic vinegar for dipping.

Tender Barley Cornbread

You can whip up this high-fiber, low-fat cornbread fast, and it bakes in 15 minutes. Use stone-ground cornmeal if you can.

¾ cup yellow cornmeal
½ cup barley flour
⅓ cup whole wheat flour (regular or pastry flour)
2 tablespoons sugar
2 teaspoons baking powder
½ teaspoon salt
¼ teaspoon baking soda
1 cup reduced-fat soy milk
¼ cup unsweetened applesauce

Preheat the oven to 425°F. Whisk together the cornmeal, barley and whole wheat flours, sugar, baking powder, salt, and baking soda in a medium bowl. Add the soy milk and applesauce and stir just until mixed. Scrape into an 8" × 8" nonstick baking pan and smooth the top. Bake for 15 minutes. Cut the hot cornbread into 6 equal pieces.

MAKES 6 SERVINGS

Per serving: 150 calories, 4 g protein, 32 g carbohydrates, 5 g sugar, 1 g total fat, 6% calories from fat, 0 mg cholesterol, 3 g fiber, 237 mg sodium

High-Protein Oat Waffles

If you didn't make these crisp, ultra-nutritious waffles yourself, you'd never guess beans were among the ingredients. Soaking the beans takes just minutes before you retire for the night, and in the morning, you can make the batter quickly in the blender. (Note: To cook waffles without added fat, you will need a good-quality nonstick waffle iron.)

These waffles take a little longer to bake than ordinary waffles (about 8 minutes), so you may want to make them ahead of time. They can be reheated quickly in a toaster. Topped with chili or creamed vegetables, they make a great lunch or supper. For gluten-free waffles, substitute brown rice flakes or quinoa flakes for the oats.

½ cup dried cannellini, white kidney, or great Northern beans
2¼ cups water
1¾ cups old-fashioned oats
2 tablespoons sugar or 1 tablespoon agave nectar
¾ tablespoon whole flaxseed
1 tablespoon baking powder
1½ teaspoons vanilla extract, or ¾ teaspoon vanilla extract and
      ¾ teaspoon orange, almond, or coconut extract
1 teaspoon salt

The night before: Place the beans in a large bowl and cover generously with water. Refrigerate overnight or for up to a week.

In the morning: Drain the beans, discarding the soaking water. Place in a blender with 2¼ cups fresh water and the oats, nectar, flaxseed, baking powder, vanilla, and salt. Blend until smooth, light, and foamy. Set aside and preheat a nonstick waffle iron.

Pour a generous ⅓ cup of batter onto the hot waffle iron for each 4" waffle, close the iron, and cook for a minimum of 8 minutes. If the iron is hard to open, let the waffle cook for another minute or two.

Repeat with the remaining batter, blending briefly before pouring each waffle. If the batter thickens while standing, add enough water to return it to its original consistency.

The waffles should be golden brown and crisp. Serve immediately or cool completely on a rack and freeze in an airtight container. Serve with your favorite toppings.

MAKES TEN 4" WAFFLES (5 SERVINGS)

Per serving: 196 calories, 10 g protein, 35 g carbohydrates, 2 g sugar, 3 g total fat, 11% calories from fat, 0 mg cholesterol, 6 g fiber, 386 mg sodium

Wheatberry Pancakes

Who would guess that with the help of your blender, you could make deliciously light pancakes from freshly ground wheat in minutes? Try these! Leftover batter works great for waffles, too.

- 1 cups wheat berries (whole wheat kernels)
- 1 tablespoon whole flaxseed
- 2 cups water
- ⅓ cup chickpea flour (besan) or low–fat soy flour
- 1 tablespoon sugar
- 2 teaspoons lemon juice
- 2 teaspoons baking powder
- ½ teaspoon baking soda
- ½ teaspoon salt

Place the wheat berries, flaxseed, and water in a blender and process at high speed for about 2 minutes. Add the flour and process for 2 to 3 minutes or until very smooth. Add the sugar, lemon juice, baking powder, baking soda, and salt and process until well mixed.

Heat a heavy nonstick griddle or skillet (a nonstick electric griddle cooks very evenly) over high heat until drops of water dance on the surface and then quickly disappear. Reduce the heat to medium–high. Working in batches if necessary, pour dollops of batter quickly onto the griddle, leaving space to expand. When bubbles appear on the surface, gently flip the pancakes. Don't overcook; they should be a bit puffy when you take them off the griddle, so they are light and cakey.

MAKES TWELVE 4" PANCAKES (3 SERVINGS)

Per serving: 261 calories, 11 g protein, 53 g carbohydrates, 6 g sugar, 3 g total fat, 9% calories from fat, 0 mg cholesterol, 9 g fiber, 534 mg sodium

Fruit Smoothie

This quick and easy recipe is great way to start your day—or give you a healthy boost anytime.

> ½ cup unsweetened apple or orange juice
> ½ cup reduced-fat soy milk
> ½ cup frozen blueberries or other berries
> ½ cup frozen peaches
> 1 tablespoon soy protein powder

Combine the juice, soy milk, berries, peaches, and protein powder in a blender or food processor. Blend until very smooth.

MAKES 1 SERVING

Per serving: 148 calories, 4 g protein, 32 g carbohydrates, 13 g sugar, 2 g total fat, 9% calories from fat, 0 mg cholesterol, 3 g fiber, 65 mg sodium

Dips, Spreads, and Dressings

Low-Fat Guacamole

This "mock-amole" is creamy and tasty. It is delicious with baked corn tortilla chips.

> 5 ounces fresh green beans or frozen small whole green beans
> 5 ounces frozen baby lima beans
> ½ cup reduced-fat firm or extra-firm silken tofu
> 3 tablespoons lemon juice
> 2 cloves garlic, crushed
> ¾ teaspoon salt
> ½ teaspoon ground cumin
> ¼ cup chunky no-sugar-added tomato salsa

Cook the green beans and lima beans in enough water to cover for about 5 minutes or just until tender but not mushy. Drain well, transfer to a food processor, and blend until smooth.

Add the tofu, lemon juice, garlic, salt, and cumin and blend until smooth. Add the salsa and pulse briefly to mix. Scoop into a covered bowl and refrigerate.

MAKES 2 CUPS

Per ¼ cup: 37 calories, 2 g protein, 7 g carbohydrates, 1 g sugar, 0.5 g total fat, 5% calories from fat, 0 mg cholesterol, 2 g fiber, 226 mg sodium

Vegetarian "Refried" Beans

This fat-free version of refried beans has a light texture and can be made with a variety of beans. It also makes a great warm bean dip or a delicious cold spread for sandwiches, wraps, or crackers.

  4½ cups cooked or 3 cans (15 ounces each) black, small red,
        kidney, or pinto beans, rinsed and drained
  1 small onion, finely chopped
  2 tablespoons red wine vinegar
  1 teaspoon salt
  1 teaspoon ground cumin
  1 teaspoon dried oregano
  1 teaspoon dried garlic granules
  1 teaspoon chili powder
    Hot-pepper sauce to taste (optional)
    A few dashes of liquid smoke (optional)

Place the beans, onion, vinegar, salt, cumin, oregano, garlic granules, chili powder, hot-pepper sauce, if desired, and liquid smoke, if desired, in a food processor. Blend for several minutes or until very smooth. Transfer to a serving bowl, cover, and refrigerate.

For a hot dip, microwave on high for about 3 minutes or heat in a skillet, stirring constantly.

MAKES 4 CUPS

Per ¼ cup: 68 calories, 4 g protein, 12 g carbohydrates, 0.5 g sugar, 0.5 g total fat, 4% calories from fat, 0 mg cholesterol, 4 g fiber, 120 mg sodium

Spinach Hummus

Most versions of this popular Middle Eastern chickpea dip are chock-full of olive oil and sesame tahini. This recipe contains a little tahini and plenty of spinach or other greens for good nutrition and lots of color. Serve with raw veggies and wedges of sprouted-wheat pita bread or with fat-free dark rye-crisp crackers. Heating the chickpeas before processing makes a creamier hummus.

  1 package (10 ounces) frozen spinach, thawed
  2 cups well-cooked chickpeas or 1 can (19 ounces) chickpeas, heated and drained
  ⅓ cup lemon juice
  1 tablespoon sesame tahini
4–6 cloves garlic
 1½ teaspoons salt
  1 teaspoon ground cumin
  ¼ teaspoon cayenne pepper

Squeeze as much liquid from the spinach as you can and chop with a sharp knife. Set aside.

Place the chickpeas, lemon juice, tahini, garlic, salt, cumin, and cayenne in a food processor. Blend until as smooth as desired, adding a bit of water if necessary (it will thicken somewhat in the refrigerator). Add the spinach and blend briefly.

Transfer to a serving bowl, cover with plastic wrap, and refrigerate until ready to serve.

MAKES ABOUT 3½ CUPS

Per ¼ cup: 107 calories, 7 g protein, 19 g carbohydrates, 0.5 g sugar, 2 g total fat, 13% calories from fat, 0 mg cholesterol, 6 g fiber, 336 mg sodium

Variations

Try this recipe with cooked or thawed frozen kale, Swiss chard, or collard greens instead of spinach.

For a more traditional hummus, omit the greens and decrease the salt to 1 teaspoon, the cumin to ½ teaspoon, and the cayenne to a pinch.

For delicious red pepper hummus, make the traditional hummus variation and add ½ cup drained and rinsed roasted red peppers from a jar when you process the chickpeas.

Cypriot Yellow Split Pea and Dill Spread

This easy spread is delicious with dark rye-crisp crackers or sprouted-wheat pita wedges. The garlic mellows considerably when cooked.

- 1 cup dried yellow split peas
- 7 cloves garlic
- 1 small onion, chopped
- 1 teaspoon salt
- 3 cups water
- 3 tablespoons fresh lemon juice
- 2 teaspoons dried dill weed or 2 tablespoons chopped fresh dill
  Freshly ground black pepper to taste
  Paprika (optional)
- 1 sprig fresh dill (optional)

Combine the split peas, 6 of the garlic cloves, onion, salt, and water in a medium saucepan. Bring to a boil, skimming off any foam. Reduce the heat, cover, and simmer for 30 minutes.

Transfer to a food processor or blender and process, or use a hand-held blender in the pan. (Remove the "pusher" from the top of the food processor so hot air can escape. Cover the hole loosely with a folded clean cloth while processing.) Crush the remaining garlic clove and add to the mixture along with the lemon juice and dill. Process until very smooth. Season with the pepper.

Pour into a decorative serving bowl, cover, and let cool. Garnish with the paprika and dill sprig, if desired.

This spread is best served at room temperature. If you store it in the refrigerator, simply bring it to room temperature before serving.

MAKES 2½ CUPS

Per ¼ cup: 74 calories, 5 g protein, 14 g carbohydrates, 2 g sugar, 0.5 g total fat, 2% calories from fat, 0 mg cholesterol, 5 g fiber, 193 mg sodium

Red Wine Vinaigrette

This is a good basic dressing for many types of salads. Unlike plain juice or water, the oil substitute will help the dressing stick to the greens. I like to make 2 cups at a time and refrigerate the extra.

Fat-Free Oil Substitute

- 1 cup cold water
- 1 tablespoon low-sodium vegetarian broth powder
- 2 teaspoons cornstarch

Dressing

- 1¼ cups Fat-Free Oil Substitute
- ¼ cup red wine vinegar
- 1 tablespoon balsamic vinegar
- 1 clove garlic, crushed
- 1 teaspoon salt
- 1 tablespoon Dijon mustard (optional)
- 1 tablespoon brown sugar (optional)

For the oil substitute: Place the water in a small saucepan and whisk in the broth powder and cornstarch. Cook over medium–high heat, stirring constantly, until thickened and clear.

For the dressing: Whisk, shake, or blend the oil substitute, red wine and balsamic vinegars, garlic, salt, mustard, if desired, and sugar, if desired, until well mixed. Transfer to a jar and refrigerate.

MAKES 1½ CUPS

Per 2 tablespoons: 6 calories, 0.5 g protein, 2 g carbohydrates, 0 g sugar, 0 g total fat, 0% calories from fat, 0 mg cholesterol, 0.5 g fiber, 160 mg sodium

Variation

Balsamic Vinaigrette: Omit the red wine vinegar and use 5 tablespoons balsamic vinegar. Use the optional mustard and brown sugar.

Per 2 tablespoons: 11 calories, 0.5 g protein, 3 g carbohydrates, 1 g sugar, 0.5 g total fat, 3% calories from fat, 0 mg cholesterol, 0.5 g fiber, 176 mg sodium

Spinach Dip

Serve this blender dip with raw vegetables and/or fat-free dark rye-crisp crackers.

    20 ounces reduced-fat extra-firm silken tofu
    ¼ cup lemon juice
     1 envelope Lipton Recipe Secrets Vegetable Soup Mix
    ½ teaspoon salt
     1 package (10 ounces) frozen chopped spinach, thawed and
         squeezed dry
     2 scallions, minced
     1 can (8 ounces) water chestnuts, drained and chopped
         (optional)
     1 tablespoon vegetarian bacon bits (optional)

Place the tofu, lemon juice, soup mix, and salt in a food processor and blend until smooth. Add the spinach, scallions, water chestnuts, if desired, and bacon bits, if desired, and pulse until mixed. Transfer to a serving bowl, cover, and refrigerate until ready to serve.

MAKES 4 CUPS (12 SERVINGS)

Per serving: 16 calories, 1 g protein, 3 g carbohydrates, 1 g sugar, 0.5 g total fat, 10% calories from fat, 0 mg cholesterol, 1 g fiber, 226 mg sodium

Creamy Poppy Seed Dressing

This quick and easy dressing is very low in fat. With just the right amount of sweetness, it's great on fruit salads and spinach salads.

  8　ounces reduced-fat firm or extra-firm silken tofu, crumbled
  6　ounces (½ can) frozen apple juice concentrate, thawed
  6　tablespoons reduced-fat soy milk
  3　tablespoons cider vinegar
  1　tablespoon poppy seeds
1½　tablespoons chopped onion
1½　tablespoons Dijon mustard
  1　scant teaspoon salt

Place all the ingredients in a blender and process until smooth. Transfer to a jar and refrigerate. Shake before serving.

MAKES 2 CUPS

Per ¼ cup: 45 calories, 3 g protein, 7 g carbohydrates, 1 g sugar, 1 g total fat, 18% calories from fat, 0 mg cholesterol, 0.5 g fiber, 268 mg sodium

Creamy Black Pepper Dressing

This is sure to be a favorite, especially if you are a fan of spinach salads. The blender is the key to the creamy texture.

1½　tablespoons low-sodium vegetarian broth powder
  1　package (12.3 ounces) reduced-fat firm silken tofu
  1　large clove garlic, finely chopped
  3　tablespoons fresh lemon juice
  1　tablespoon rice vinegar
  1　tablespoon nutritional yeast flakes
1½　teaspoons whole black peppercorns
  1　teaspoon miso
  1　teaspoon sugar
  ¾　teaspoon salt
  ⅔　cup water

Place all the ingredients in a blender and process until very smooth. Transfer to a jar and refrigerate. Shake well before serving.

MAKES 2 CUPS

Per 2 tablespoons: 15 calories, 2 g protein, 2 g carbohydrates, 0.5 g sugar, 0.5 g total fat, 11% calories from fat, 0 mg cholesterol, 0.5 g fiber, 123 mg sodium

Soups

Dutch Green Pea Soup

A very satisfying meal on a cold day! Serve this soup hot along with dark pumpernickel bread.

    1   cup green split peas
    8   cups low-sodium vegetarian broth
    1   tablespoon vegetarian bacon bits
    2   medium new or red potatoes, peeled and chopped
    2   medium leeks, chopped, including any tender green parts
    ½   cup chopped celery, including leaves
    ½   teaspoon dried savory
    ½   teaspoon liquid smoke
    1   package (10–12 ounces) low-fat vegetarian hot dogs or
            sausages, sliced diagonally into chunks
        Salt to taste
        Freshly ground black pepper to taste

Bring the split peas, broth, and bacon bits to a boil in a large saucepan, skimming off any foam. Reduce the heat, cover, and simmer for about 3 hours. Add the potatoes, leeks, celery, savory, liquid smoke, and hot dogs or sausages. Simmer for 30 minutes or until the potatoes are tender. Season with the salt and pepper.

MAKES 8 SERVINGS

Per serving: 184 calories, 15 g protein, 27 g carbohydrates, 3 g sugar, 3 g total fat, 11% calories from fat, 0 mg cholesterol, 7 g fiber, 36 mg sodium

Barley and Winter Squash Chowder

This is a lovely soup for a cold evening.

    4   cups low-sodium vegetarian broth
    1   pound winter squash, peeled, seeded, and cut into ¾" cubes
    ½   large onion, chopped
    6   ounces low-fat chicken substitute strips, such as Butler Soy
            Curls, reconstituted
    ¾   cup pearled barley
    8   ounces red potatoes, chopped
    ¼   cup chopped celery leaves and tops
    1½ teaspoons vegetarian bacon bits
    1   bay leaf
    ½   teaspoon dried thyme
    ½   teaspoon dried savory
    1½ cups reduced-fat soy milk
        Salt to taste
        Freshly ground black pepper to taste
        Chopped fresh parsley (optional)

Place the broth, squash, onion, chicken substitute strips, barley, potatoes, celery, bacon bits, bay leaf, thyme, and savory in a soup pot and
bring to a boil. Reduce the heat to low, cover, and simmer for 30 minutes. Remove the bay leaf, stir in the soy milk, and season with the salt
and pepper. Sprinkle each serving with chopped parsley, if desired.

MAKES 6 SERVINGS

Per serving: 204 calories, 11 g protein, 40 g carbohydrates, 4 g sugar, 1 g total fat, 4%
calories from fat, 0 mg cholesterol, 8 g fiber, 229 mg sodium

Creamy Mushroom Bisque

A food processor turns this dairy-free soup into a rich, creamy treat
with a delightful mushroom flavor.

    1   small onion, finely chopped
    5   cups mushroom broth

  1 bay leaf
  ½ teaspoon dried thyme
  ⅔ cup old-fashioned oats
 12 ounces mushrooms, sliced
  2 teaspoons low-sodium soy sauce
  2 tablespoons dry sherry (optional)
     Salt to taste
     Freshly ground black pepper to taste
     Vegan Parmesan cheese (optional)

Steam-fry the onion in a heavy nonstick skillet over medium heat until soft but not browned, adding very small amounts of water as needed to prevent sticking and burning. (Or place in a microwaveable dish, cover, and microwave on high for 3 minutes.)

Place the broth, bay leaf, thyme, and oats in a medium saucepan. Add the onion and bring to a boil, then reduce the heat to low, cover, and simmer for 20 minutes or until the oats are soft.

Meanwhile, steam-fry the mushrooms in a large, heavy nonstick skillet over high heat, adding a sprinkle of salt and very small amounts of water as needed to prevent sticking and burning. Cook until the mushrooms release and reabsorb their liquid. Remove from the heat and set aside.

When the oats are soft, remove the bay leaf and puree the soup until creamy with a hand-held blender or in batches in a blender or food processor. (Remove the middle part of the blender or food processor's lid so hot air can escape. Cover the hole loosely with a folded clean cloth while blending.)

Return the soup to the pan and add the mushrooms, soy sauce, sherry (if desired), salt, pepper, and vegan Parmesan (if desired). Serve hot.

MAKES 4 SERVINGS

Per serving: 80 calories, 5 g protein, 14 g carbohydrates, 3 g sugar, 1 g total fat, 12% calories from fat, 0 mg cholesterol, 3 g fiber, 93 mg sodium

Black-Eyed Pea and Sweet Potato Soup

This delectable soup contains Southern ingredients—black-eyed peas, vegetarian bacon and sausage, sweet potatoes, and greens.

    1 large onion, chopped
    3 cloves garlic, minced
    6 cups low-sodium vegetarian broth
    ¼ cup tomato paste
    3 cups cooked or 2 cans (15 ounces each) black-eyed peas,
         rinsed and drained
    2 tablespoons vegetarian bacon bits or a few dashes of liquid
         smoke
    2 teaspoons dried oregano
    1 bay leaf
    ½ teaspoon salt
    ½ teaspoon crushed red pepper
    4 ounces kale, collards, or other dark greens, cleaned, trimmed,
         and thinly sliced
    1 pound sweet potatoes, peeled and chopped
    2 vegetarian Italian sausages, such as Lightlife Smart Links
         Italian or Yves Veggie Spicy Italian Sausage, cut into ¼"
         slices

Steam-fry the onion and garlic in a large, heavy nonstick skillet over medium heat until soft, adding very small amounts of water as needed to prevent sticking and burning. (Or place in a microwaveable dish, cover, and microwave on high for 5 minutes.)

Place the broth, tomato paste, black-eyed peas, bacon bits or liquid smoke, oregano, bay leaf, salt, red pepper, greens, sweet potatoes, and sausage in a large saucepan. Add the onion and garlic and simmer for 30 minutes or until the sweet potatoes are tender. Remove the bay leaf and serve immediately.

MAKES 6 SERVINGS

Per serving: 257 calories, 16 g protein, 44 g carbohydrates, 8 g sugar, 3 g total fat, 10% calories from fat, 0 mg cholesterol, 10 g fiber, 263 mg sodium

Red Lentil and Sweet Potato Soup

This hearty soup makes a great light lunch or a starter for a several-course meal. Blending gives it a delightfully smooth texture.

2 small onions, chopped
½ teaspoon ground cumin
½ teaspoon ground ginger
4 cups low-sodium vegetarian broth
2 cups cubed peeled sweet potatoes
⅔ cup red or pink lentils, rinsed
1 teaspoon lemon juice
¼ teaspoon salt
   White pepper to taste
   Paprika

Steam-fry the onions in a large, heavy nonstick skillet over medium heat until soft, adding very small amounts of water as needed to prevent sticking and burning. (Or place in a microwaveable dish, cover, and microwave on high for 5 minutes.) Stir in the cumin and ginger and blend well.

Place the broth, sweet potatoes, and lentils in a medium soup pot. Add the onions and simmer, uncovered, for about 30 minutes or until the lentils are tender. Add the lemon juice, salt, and white pepper. Process using a hand-held blender in the pan or in batches in a blender or food processor, until creamy. (Remove the middle part of the blender or food processor lid so hot air can escape. Cover the hole loosely with a folded clean cloth while blending.) Serve hot and with paprika sprinkled on top of each bowl.

MAKES 4 SERVINGS

Per serving: 185 calories, 10 g protein, 36 g carbohydrates, 4 g sugar, 1 g total fat, 3% calories from fat, 0 mg cholesterol, 6 g fiber, 158 mg sodium

Sandwiches and Salads

Black Bean Soft Tacos

In Mexico, tacos are usually made with fresh, hot tortillas (not deep-fried ones). This machine-blended filling brings you all the traditional taste and heartiness of the real thing.

Tofu Sour Cream

- 1 package (12.3 ounces) reduced-fat extra-firm silken tofu, crumbled
- 3 tablespoons lemon juice
- ½ teaspoon sugar
- ¼ teaspoon salt

Tacos

- 8 corn tortillas (6")
- 1½ cups Vegetarian "Refried" Beans made with black beans (page 199)
- 2 cups (1 recipe) Low-Fat Guacamole (page 198)
- 1 cup no-sugar-added tomato salsa
- 4 cups finely shredded green cabbage or lettuce
- 1 cup Tofu Sour Cream

For the tofu sour cream: Place the tofu, lemon juice, sugar, and salt in a food processor or blender and process until very smooth. Refrigerate in a covered container for up to 1 week.

For the tacos: Heat the tortillas (see Note). Spread about 3 tablespoons of beans down the middle of each tortilla. Top with guacamole, salsa, cabbage or lettuce, and tofu sour cream. Eat out of hand with lots of napkins!

Note: If the tortillas are frozen, heat them between two microwaveable plates on high for about 1 minute, then turn over the plates and heat for 1 minute longer. You can soften thawed or fresh tortillas in a hot, dry pan; grill them quickly just until soft; or wrap them in a clean kitchen towel moistened with hot water, then wrap them in foil and place them in the oven until all are heated. Or, wrap the tortillas in a clean kitchen towel moistened with hot water, wrap them in foil, and bake them in a 350°F oven for about 12 minutes.

If you have a noninsulated microwaveable steamer, place a little hot water under the steamer tray. Wrap the thawed tortillas in a clean kitchen towel and place them in the steamer tray. Cover and microwave for 2 to 3 minutes for 6 tortillas or 4 minutes for 12 tortillas. If you leave the wrapped tortillas in the steamer, they will stay hot during the meal.

MAKES 8 SERVINGS

Per serving: 174 calories, 10 g protein, 33 g carbohydrates, 3 g sugar, 1 g total fat, 7% calories from fat, 0 mg cholesterol, 7 g fiber, 557 mg sodium

Asparagus and Veggie Ham Panini

This Italian panini will become a lunchtime favorite.

- 2 slices rye or sprouted-grain bread
- 2 tablespoons Tofu Mayonnaise (page 220)
- 6 thin asparagus spears, steamed or roasted
- 6 fresh basil leaves
- 2 slices low-fat vegetarian bacon or ham, such as Yves Veggie Canadian Bacon

Spread each bread slice on 1 side with 1 tablespoon tofu mayonnaise and assemble the sandwich with the rest of the ingredients the way you like it, being careful not to overfill.

The easiest way to make panini is with an electric nonstick panini press or closed indoor grill. Set the timer for 5 minutes, then check the bread. If it is not as golden and crisp as you like, cook for a few minutes longer. Cut the sandwich into triangles and serve hot.

If you do not have a panini press or grill, cook the sandwich in a heavy nonstick skillet or on a griddle over medium heat, placing a flat heavy lid on the sandwich as you brown each side.

Per serving (using rye bread): 308 calories, 31 g protein, 32 g carbohydrates, 0.2 g sugar, 4 g total fat, 11% calories from fat, 0 mg cholesterol, 6 g fiber, 825 mg sodium

Italian Stuffed Griddle Dumplings (Consum)

This traditional "griddle dumpling" from Romagna is actually a stuffed Italian flatbread, similar to a calzone but stuffed with greens. This easy version uses whole wheat pitas.

    6 whole wheat pitas
    ½ pound Swiss chard, beet greens, spinach, or savoy cabbage, or
          a mixture
    ½ pound bitter greens, such as arugula, radicchio, rapini,
          Chinese broccoli, mustard or turnip greens, or curly endive
  1½ teaspoons chopped garlic
    ¼ cup low-sodium vegetarian broth
    ¼ teaspoon salt, and extra to taste
       Freshly ground black pepper to taste

Cut the pitas in half and open to form a pocket. Wash, trim, and thinly slice the greens.

Place the garlic, broth, greens, and salt in a large, deep nonstick skillet. Bring to a boil, then cover, reduce the heat to medium, and cook until tender. If any liquid remains, uncover and cook over high heat, stirring constantly, until it evaporates. Season with the salt and pepper and set aside to cool.

Drain the greens and stuff inside the pita halves. Heat the filled pitas on a hot, dry griddle or cast-iron pan over high heat, turning frequently, until hot and flecked with brown spots. Serve hot.

MAKES 6 SERVINGS

Per serving: 188 calories, 8 g protein, 38 g carbohydrates, 2 g sugar, 2 g total fat, 8% calories from fat, 0 mg cholesterol, 6 g fiber, 510 mg sodium

Mediterranean Veggie Panini

Italian sandwich making has become an art form in the northern city of Milan and has spread all over Europe and North America. Sandwich bars in Italy range from humble places to the height of sophistication, and some offer as many as 30 varieties.

> 2 slices rye or sprouted-grain bread, such as Ezekiel Bread
> 2 tablespoons fat-free Italian vinaigrette dressing
> 2 jarred roasted red peppers, rinsed and patted dry
> 1 cup tender kale leaves or other greens
> 2 small firm, ripe tomatoes, sliced (fresh Roma tomatoes are best because they are not overly juicy)
> ½ cup sliced marinated artichoke hearts, rinsed, drained, and patted dry

Moisten each bread slice on 1 side with 1 tablespoon dressing and assemble the sandwich with the rest of the ingredients the way you like it, being careful not to overfill.

The easiest way to make panini is with an electric nonstick panini press or closed indoor grill. Set the timer for 5 minutes, then check the bread. If it is not as golden and crisp as you like, cook for a few minutes longer. Cut the sandwich into triangles and serve hot.

If you do not have a panini press or grill, cook the sandwich in a heavy nonstick skillet or on a griddle over medium heat, placing a flat heavy lid on the sandwich as you brown each side.

MAKES 1 SERVING

Per serving (using rye bread): 311 calories, 13 g protein, 49 g carbohydrates, 4.9 g sugar, 3 g total fat, 8% calories from fat, 0 mg cholesterol, 13.3 g fiber, 849 mg sodium

Sloppy Joes for Two

Here's a tasty and healthful version of an old favorite.

½ small onion, finely chopped
½ small green bell pepper, cored, seeded, and chopped
½ small red bell pepper, cored, seeded, and chopped
6 medium mushrooms, chopped
¾ cup low-fat vegetarian hamburger crumbles
½ cup fat-free barbecue sauce, such as Bull's-Eye Original
1 tablespoon tomato paste dissolved in ½ cup hot water
2 sprouted-wheat hamburger buns, such as Alvarado Street
      Bakery buns, split and toasted

Steam-fry the onions, peppers, and mushrooms in a heavy nonstick skillet over high heat until softened, adding water by the tablespoon as needed to prevent sticking and burning.

Add the hamburger crumbles, barbecue sauce, and tomato paste mixture. Cook, stirring, until the sauce is the desired consistency. Spoon over the split buns or fill them like a sandwich.

MAKES 2 SERVINGS

Per serving: 218 calories, 14 g protein, 40 g carbohydrates, 11 g sugar, 2 g total fat, 7% calories from fat, 0 mg cholesterol, 6 g fiber, 508 mg sodium

Orange Quinoa and Bulgur Tabbouleh

This is a delicious and unusual version of the well-known Middle Eastern salad.

½ cup medium-grain bulgur wheat
1½ cups water
½ cup quinoa
¾ cup Fat-Free Oil Substitute (page 202)
¼ cup lemon juice
1 teaspoon salt
1 teaspoon ground coriander

2 pinches ground cinnamon
  Freshly ground black pepper to taste
2 cups chopped fresh parsley
1 cup cooked or canned black-eyed peas, rinsed and drained
⅔ cup chopped, seeded green bell pepper
½ cup chopped fresh mint or lemon balm
½ cup chopped scallion
  Grated peel of 2 oranges
4 jarred roasted red peppers, rinsed and chopped
  Orange wedges (optional)
  Mint, parsley, or lemon balm sprigs (optional)

Soak the bulgur in ½ cup boiling water in a large bowl, covered, for 30 minutes. Meanwhile, bring the quinoa and 1 cup water to a boil in a small saucepan. Reduce the heat to low, cover, and cook for 15 minutes. Remove from the heat and let stand until the bulgur is ready.

Whisk or blend together the oil substitute, lemon juice, salt, coriander, cinnamon, and black pepper in a small bowl. Set aside.

Combine the quinoa with the bulgur. Add the parsley, black-eyed peas, bell pepper, mint or lemon balm, scallion, orange peel, red peppers, and oil dressing and mix well. Garnish with orange wedges and sprigs of mint, parsley, or lemon balm, if desired. Refrigerate, but let stand at room temperature for 30 minutes before serving.

MAKES 8 SERVINGS

Per serving: 136 calories, 5 g protein, 29 g carbohydrates, 2 g sugar, 1 g total fat, 7% calories from fat, 0 mg cholesterol, 7 g fiber, 303 mg sodium

Cherry Tomato and Brown Rice Salad with Artichoke Hearts

This delicious salad is a complete meal and a great picnic or potluck dish. Because neither tomatoes nor rice benefit from refrigeration, it should be served at room temperature.

    3 cups cooked brown basmati rice, warm
    6 ounces marinated artichoke hearts, rinsed in hot water,
        drained, and sliced
    1 cup chopped scallions
 1½ pounds red, yellow, or mixed cherry tomatoes, halved
    ½ cup chopped fresh basil
    ½ cup fat-free Italian dressing
    3 tablespoons lemon juice
    2 cloves garlic, crushed
    ¼ teaspoon salt
      Freshly ground black pepper to taste
    1 head crisp lettuce

Place the rice in a large salad bowl and add the artichokes, scallions, tomatoes, and basil. Mix gently.

Combine the Italian dressing, lemon juice, garlic, salt, and pepper in a small bowl or jar. Whisk or shake until well blended. Pour over the salad and mix gently. Serve on beds of lettuce on individual plates.

MAKES 6 SERVINGS

Per serving: 153 calories, 4 g protein, 32 g carbohydrates, 3 g sugar, 1 g total fat, 6% calories from fat, 0 mg cholesterol, 4 g fiber, 376 mg sodium

Thai-Style Coleslaw

This easy coleslaw makes a great winter accompaniment to an Asian meal or spices up any other meal.

3   cups finely shredded green or savoy cabbage
1   medium carrot, shredded
1   small sweet onion, thinly sliced
2   tablespoons minced fresh mint or 2 teaspoons dried mint
2   tablespoons minced fresh cilantro, basil, or parsley
2   tablespoons low-sodium soy sauce
2   tablespoons lime juice
2   tablespoons water
1   tablespoon sugar
1   tablespoon grated lime peel
1½ teaspoons toasted sesame seeds

Combine the cabbage, carrot, onion, mint, and cilantro, basil, or parsley in a serving bowl.

Combine the soy sauce, lime juice, water, sugar, and lime peel in a small bowl. Pour over the salad, mix well, and refrigerate until ready to serve. Sprinkle with the sesame seeds before serving.

MAKES 4 SERVINGS

Per serving: 61 calories, 2 g protein, 13 g carbohydrates, 8 g sugar, 1 g total fat, 10% calories from fat, 0 mg cholesterol, 3 g fiber, 334 mg sodium

Red Cabbage Slaw with Cranberries and Apples

This is a very easy, attractive, and delicious make-ahead salad for winter holiday meals. A blender makes the vinaigrette in a jiffy.

Cranberry-Orange Vinaigrette
¾ cup Fat-Free Oil Substitute (page 202)
½ cup orange juice
⅓ cup chopped fresh or frozen cranberries
2 tablespoons red wine vinegar
1½ tablespoons chopped chives or scallion
1 tablespoon balsamic vinegar
1 tablespoon lemon juice
1 tablespoon sugar
1 large clove garlic, crushed
1 teaspoon salt
Freshly ground black pepper to taste

Salad
1½ pounds red cabbage, thinly sliced (about 5 cups)
¾ cup fresh or frozen cranberries
2 crisp sweet apples, sliced

For the vinaigrette: Blend the oil substitute, orange juice, cranberries, wine vinegar, chives or scallion, balsamic vinegar, lemon juice, sugar, garlic, salt, and pepper in a blender. If making ahead, transfer to a covered container and refrigerate.

For the salad: Combine the cabbage, cranberries, and vinaigrette in a medium salad bowl and toss gently. Cover and refrigerate for at least 2 hours to allow the flavors to blend. When ready to serve, slice the apples (with peel), add to the salad, and toss well.

MAKES 8 SERVINGS

Per serving: 70 calories, 1 g protein, 18 g carbohydrates, 11 g sugar, 0.5 g total fat, 2% calories from fat, 0 mg cholesterol, 3 g fiber, 251 mg sodium

Sautéed Portobello Mushroom Salad

This is a very simple and delicious salad for two.

- 8 cups cleaned mixed baby salad greens
- ¼ cup Fat-Free Oil Substitute (page 202)
- 2 tablespoons balsamic vinegar
- 1 teaspoon Dijon mustard
- ¼ teaspoon salt
- ¼ teaspoon coarsely ground black pepper
- 2 large portobello mushrooms
  Wine or vegetable broth
- 4 scallions, sliced

Divide the greens between two serving plates. In a small bowl, whisk together the oil substitute, vinegar, mustard, salt, and pepper. Set aside.

Remove the stems from the mushrooms and scrape away the dark gills with the edge of a spoon.

Heat a large, heavy nonstick skillet over high heat and add the mushrooms. Cover and cook until slightly browned on the bottoms and beginning to release a bit of liquid. Add a very small amount of wine or broth as needed to prevent sticking. Turn the mushrooms and brown the other side.

Quickly slice the mushrooms and place them evenly over the greens. Drizzle with the dressing, sprinkle with the scallions, and serve immediately.

MAKES 2 SERVINGS

Per serving: 95 calories, 7 g protein, 19 g carbohydrates, 4 g sugar, 1 g total fat, 6% calories from fat, 0 mg cholesterol, 7 g fiber, 308 mg sodium

BLT Salad

A salad version of the well-loved sandwich that uses a handy mayonnaise substitute. Cooks, plug in your blenders!

Tofu Mayonnaise
     1   package (12.3 ounces) reduced-fat extra-firm silken tofu
     2   tablespoons cider vinegar or lemon juice
  1⅛   teaspoons salt
     ½   teaspoon dry mustard
     ⅛   teaspoon white pepper

Salad
     6   cups torn romaine lettuce
     6   cups cubed sprouted-wheat bread, lightly toasted
     4   slices low-fat vegetarian bacon, such as Yves Veggie Canadian
          Bacon or Lightlife Fakin' Bacon
     2   cups chopped ripe firm tomatoes
     2   scallions, sliced
     ½   cup cider vinegar
     ⅓   cup Fat-Free Oil Substitute (page 202)
     ¼   cup Tofu Mayonnaise
     5   teaspoons sugar
          Freshly ground black pepper to taste

For the mayonnaise: Combine the tofu, vinegar or lemon juice, salt, mustard, and pepper in a food processor or blender (or place the ingredients in a medium bowl and use a hand-held blender) and process until very smooth. It will keep in a covered container in the refrigerator for about 2 weeks.

For the salad: Combine the lettuce, bread cubes, bacon, tomatoes, and scallions in a large bowl.

Whisk together the vinegar, oil substitute, tofu mayonnaise, sugar, and pepper in a medium bowl until well blended. Toss with the salad. Divide the salad evenly among 4 salad bowls or plates and serve immediately.

MAKES 4 SERVINGS

Per serving: 259 calories, 13 g protein, 42 g carbohydrates, 11 g sugar, 2 g total fat, 8% calories from fat, 0 mg cholesterol, 10 g fiber, 639 mg sodium

Main Courses

Balkan-Style Slow-Cooker Stew

Balkan cooking is similar to Greek cuisine. Serve with toasted sprouted-wheat bread or buns for dipping.

    3 large onions, sliced
    3 cloves garlic, minced
    4 large red, yellow, green, or mixed bell peppers, sliced into
         thin strips
   12 ounces low-fat chicken substitute strips, such as Yves Veggie
         Chicken Tenders or Lightlife Smart Menu Chik'n Strips
    1 can (14 ounces) low-sodium diced tomatoes
    1 small dried red chile pepper, seeded
    ½ teaspoon ground cloves
    ½ teaspoon ground cinnamon
    ¼ teaspoon ground allspice
    2 cups low-sodium vegetarian broth
       Salt to taste
       Freshly ground black pepper to taste

Heat a large, heavy nonstick skillet over high heat. Add the onions, garlic, and bell peppers. Steam-fry until the onion softens, adding very small amounts of water as needed to prevent sticking and burning.

Place the chicken substitute strips in a slow cooker and spoon the cooked vegetables on top. Stir in the tomatoes (with juice), chile pepper, cloves, cinnamon, allspice, and broth. Cook on high for 3 hours. Season with the salt and black pepper.

MAKES 4 SERVINGS

Per serving: 185 calories, 19 g protein, 30 g carbohydrates, 12 g sugar, 1 g total fat, 2% calories from fat, 0 mg cholesterol, 9 g fiber, 550 mg sodium

White Bean and Sweet Potato Stew

All you need is whole grain bread to go with this Italian-inspired stew.

　1　large onion, chopped
　4　cloves garlic, chopped
　3　cups cooked or 2 cans (15 ounces each) cannellini, white
　　　kidney, or great Northern beans, rinsed and drained
　1　can (28 ounces) low-sodium diced tomatoes
　1　pound sweet potatoes, peeled and chopped
　12　ounces kale, stripped from stalks, washed, thinly sliced, and
　　　briefly steamed
　8　ounces cremini mushrooms, sliced
　½　cup low-sodium vegetarian broth
　½　cup dry red wine (can be nonalcoholic) or ¼ cup dry sherry
　1　tablespoon vegetarian bacon bits
　1　teaspoon salt
　1　teaspoon dried rosemary
　1　teaspoon dried thyme
　1　teaspoon dried basil
　1　bay leaf
　¼　teaspoon crushed red pepper
　　　Salt to taste
　　　Freshly ground black pepper to taste

Steam-fry the onion and garlic in a large, heavy nonstick skillet over medium heat until soft, adding very small amounts of water, wine, or broth as needed to prevent sticking and burning. (Or place in a microwaveable dish, cover, and microwave on high power for 5 minutes.)

Combine the onions and garlic with the beans, tomatoes (with juice), sweet potatoes, kale, mushrooms, broth, wine, bacon bits, salt, rosemary, thyme, basil, bay leaf, and red pepper in a slow cooker. Cook on low for 6 to 7 hours or on high for 3 to 4 hours. Remove the bay leaf and season with the salt and pepper.

MAKES 6 SERVINGS

Per serving: 257 calories, 14 g protein, 50 g carbohydrates, 9 g sugar, 2 g total fat, 4% calories from fat, 0 mg cholesterol, 12 g fiber, 418 mg sodium

Lebanese-Style Lentils and Pasta

This delicious Lebanese dish makes a full meal.

        5   cups low-sodium vegetarian broth
        1   cup uncooked brown lentils, rinsed
        2   medium onions, chopped
        2   cloves garlic, chopped
        1   teaspoon ground cumin
        4   cups chopped chard, kale, or other greens or 1 package
                (10 ounces) frozen chopped spinach, thawed and
                squeezed dry
        4   ounces spaghetti or spaghettini (preferably whole wheat),
                broken into 4"-long pieces
       ¼   cup chopped fresh parsley or cilantro (optional)
            Pinch of cayenne pepper
        2   tablespoons lemon juice
            Salt to taste
            Freshly ground black pepper to taste

Bring the broth and lentils to a boil in a medium saucepan. Reduce the heat to low, cover, and cook for about 25 minutes or until the lentils are tender but still hold their shape.

Steam-fry the onions, garlic, and cumin in a large, heavy nonstick saucepan, stir-fry pan, or deep skillet until soft, adding very small amounts of water as needed to prevent sticking and burning. (Or place in a microwaveable dish, cover, and microwave on high for 7 minutes.)

Pour the lentils and broth into the pan with the onions. Add the greens, pasta, parsley or cilantro, if desired, and cayenne. Bring to a boil, then reduce the heat to medium. Cook, uncovered, for about 10 minutes or until the pasta is tender and most of the broth has been absorbed, leaving a sauce. Add the lemon juice and mix well. Season with the salt and black pepper. Serve hot.

MAKES 4 SERVINGS

Per serving: 318 calories, 20 g protein, 61 g carbohydrates, 7 g sugar, 1 g total fat, 3% calories from fat, 0 mg cholesterol, 17 g fiber, 204 mg sodium

Lemon and Artichoke Tagine (Moroccan Stew)

Serve this delicious stew with Bulgur Wheat and Quinoa Pilaf (page 234).

     2 tablespoons whole wheat flour
    12 ounces low-fat chicken substitute strips, such as Yves Veggie
         Chicken Tenders, Lightlife Smart Menu Chik'n Strips, or
         Morningstar Farms Meal Starters Chik'n Strips
     1 large onion, sliced
     6 cloves garlic, chopped
     2 cups sliced mushrooms
     1 large green or red bell pepper, cored, seeded, and cut into
         chunks
     2 cups low-sodium vegetarian broth
     1 tablespoon ground coriander
     1 tablespoon dried parsley
    ½ teaspoon black pepper
    ¼ teaspoon ground turmeric
    ¼ teaspoon ground ginger
    ¼ teaspoon paprika
    ¼ teaspoon crushed red pepper
     1 lemon, with peel, sliced and seeded
     1 jar (7 ounces) marinated artichoke heart quarters, rinsed
         under hot water and drained
        Salt to taste

Place the flour in a shallow dish and roll the chicken substitute strips to coat. Place the strips in a large, heavy, deep nonstick skillet or stir-fry pan over medium-high heat and cook until browned. Remove from the pan and set aside.

Add the onion and garlic to the skillet and steam-fry until soft, adding very small amounts of water as needed to prevent sticking and burning. (Or place in a microwaveable dish, cover, and microwave on high for 7 minutes.)

Add the strips, mushrooms, bell pepper, broth, coriander, parsley, black pepper, turmeric, ginger, paprika, and red pepper. Place the lemon slices on top of the stew, cover, reduce the heat, and simmer for 30 minutes.

Remove and discard the lemon slices. Stir in the artichokes and cook just until heated. Season with the salt and serve immediately.

MAKES 4 SERVINGS

Per serving: 165 calories, 20 g protein, 25 g carbohydrates, 3 g sugar, 1 g total fat, 3% calories from fat, 0 mg cholesterol, 10 g fiber, 584 mg sodium

Pasta with Lentil Marinara Sauce

Red wine (which can be a nonalcoholic variety) lends a rich flavor to this sauce, which is ready in the time it takes to cook the pasta.

- 1 pound pasta of choice
- 1 jar (26 ounces) fat-free low-sodium tomato-based pasta sauce
- 1 can (15 ounces) lentils, rinsed and drained
- ½ cup dry red wine (can be nonalcoholic) or low-sodium vegetarian broth
  Salt to taste
  Freshly ground black pepper

Cook the pasta according to package directions, then drain.

Meanwhile, combine the pasta sauce, lentils, and wine or broth in a medium saucepan. Heat gently and season with the salt and pepper. Serve over the pasta.

MAKES 5 SERVINGS

Per serving: 470 calories, 19 g protein, 91 g carbohydrates, 9 g sugar, 2 g total fat, 3% calories from fat, 0 mg cholesterol, 8 g fiber, 173 mg sodium

Vegetarian Mixed-Bean Chili Express

Healthy in a Hurry

This chili is an absolutely delicious savory treat. Serve it with brown basmati rice, sprouted-grain bread or buns, corn or sprouted-wheat tortillas, soft fresh polenta or cornbread, and a salad. Leftovers freeze well.

    6 cloves garlic, minced or crushed
    1 tablespoon chili powder (preferably a dark variety, such as
         ancho)
    1 tablespoon dried oregano
 1½ teaspoons ground cumin
   ½ teaspoon crushed red pepper
    1 can (28 ounces) low-sodium diced tomatoes
 1½ cups cooked or 1 can (15 ounces) pinto beans, rinsed and
         drained
 1½ cups cooked or 1 can (15 ounces) black beans, rinsed and
         drained
 1½ cups cooked or 1 can (15 ounces) small red or red kidney
         beans, rinsed and drained
    3 cups hot water
 1½ cups dry textured vegetable protein
    1 cup frozen whole-kernel corn
    1 large green bell pepper, cored, seeded, and chopped
   ¼ cup low-sodium soy sauce
    1 tablespoon hot-pepper sauce
    1 tablespoon onion powder
    1 tablespoon unsweetened cocoa powder
    1 teaspoon sugar
    2 tablespoons cornmeal or masa harina
       Salt to taste

Steam-fry the garlic in a large, heavy nonstick skillet for 2 minutes. Add the chili powder, oregano, cumin, and red pepper and stir-fry for 1 minute. Add the tomatoes (with juice), beans, hot water, vegetable protein, corn, bell pepper, soy sauce, hot-pepper sauce, onion powder, cocoa, and sugar. Bring to a boil, then reduce the heat, cover, and simmer for 15 to 30 minutes. During the last 5 minutes of cooking, sprinkle the cornmeal or masa harina over the top and stir in thoroughly. Season with the salt.

MAKES 6 SERVINGS

Per serving: 329 calories, 26 g protein, 57 g carbohydrates, 7 g sugar, 2 g total fat, 4% calories from fat, 0 mg cholesterol, 16 g fiber, 457 mg sodium

Black-Eyed Peas with Sweet Potatoes and Greens

A wonderful combination of flavors! Serve with brown rice or fat-free cornbread, with hot sauce on the side.

    1 package (10 ounces) frozen kale, chard, or collard greens
    4 cups low-sodium vegetarian broth
    2 packages (10 ounces each) frozen black-eyed peas, thawed and
          drained
    2 cloves garlic, minced
    1 can (18 ounces) vacuum-packed unsweetened sweet potatoes,
          drained, rinsed, and chopped, or 2 cups cooked
       A few dashes of liquid smoke

Thaw the greens in the microwave or a bowl of boiling water and drain. Chop and combine with the broth, black-eyed peas, garlic, sweet potatoes, and liquid smoke in a large saucepan. Bring to a boil, stirring often, then reduce the heat and simmer for 20 to 30 minutes.

MAKES 4 SERVINGS

Per serving: 412 calories, 32 g protein, 74 g carbohydrates, 1 g sugar, 4 g total fat, 8% calories from fat, 0 mg cholesterol, 22 g fiber, 127 mg sodium

Indonesian-Style Stir-Fried Pasta (Bamie)

This dish has just the right exotic touch.

  1 pound soy vermicelli pasta
  1 medium onion, chopped
  6 cloves garlic, minced
½–1 teaspoon crushed red pepper
  2 cups shredded napa or savoy cabbage
  2 stalks celery, sliced thinly on the diagonal
  ¼ cup water
  6 ounces low-fat beef substitute strips, such as Yves Veggie Beef Tenders, Lightlife Smart Menu Steak-Style Strips, or Morningstar Farms Meal Starters Steak Strips
  ½ cup low-sodium vegetarian broth
  ¼ cup low-sodium soy sauce
  ¾ tablespoon maple syrup
  ¾ tablespoon dark molasses
  2 teaspoons cornstarch
  1 tablespoon cold water
  4 scallions, sliced thinly on the diagonal

Cook the pasta in a large pot of boiling water until tender. Drain in a colander.

In a large, heavy nonstick wok or a skillet lightly coated with oil or cooking spray, steam-fry the onion, garlic, and red pepper for 1 minute, adding very small amounts of water as needed to prevent sticking and burning.

Add the cabbage, celery, and ¼ cup water. Cover and cook over high heat for about 3 minutes. Add the beef substitute strips and stir-fry for about 1 minute.

Combine the broth, soy sauce, maple syrup, molasses, cornstarch, and cold water in a small bowl. Stir into the pan and cook, stirring, over high heat until it thickens and boils.

Add the drained pasta and toss well with the sauce. Top with the scallions and serve.

MAKES 6 SERVINGS

Per serving: 338 calories, 10 g protein, 74 g carbohydrates, 19 g sugar, 1 g total fat, 2% calories from fat, 0 mg cholesterol, 5 g fiber, 505 mg sodium

Quick Spinach Lasagna

Although it takes a little more than an hour to make this dish, most of that is cooking time; prep takes just a few minutes.

  1 package (10 ounces) frozen spinach, thawed
  1 pound reduced-fat firm tofu
  1 tablespoon chopped or minced garlic
  1 teaspoon salt
  1 jar (26 ounces) fat-free low-sodium tomato-based pasta sauce
  1 pound whole wheat lasagna noodles
 10 button mushrooms, sliced, or 1 cup other vegetable of choice
  ¼ cup vegan Parmesan or nutritional yeast flakes

Preheat the oven to 325°F.

Combine the spinach, tofu, garlic, and salt in a medium bowl.

Coat the bottom of a 9" × 13" baking pan with tomato sauce, then add a layer of lasagna noodles, overlapping them slightly. Spread half of the spinach mixture over the noodles. Follow with another layer of noodles, then tomato sauce, and a layer of mushrooms or other veggies. Repeat until the layers reach the top of the pan. The final layer should be sauce topped with vegan Parmesan or yeast flakes.

Cover tightly with foil and bake for 1 hour. Stick a knife through the center of the lasagna to be sure the noodles are completely cooked. Let stand for 15 minutes, uncovered, before serving.

MAKES 8 SERVINGS

Per serving: 332 calories, 18 g protein, 5 g carbohydrates, 7 g sugar, 5 g total fat, 9% calories from fat, 0 mg cholesterol, 9 g fiber, 284 mg sodium

Recipe by Jennifer Reilly, RD

Eggplant Parmesan

This interpretation of an old favorite appeals to modern tastes, with "béchamel" sauce and vegan Parmesan providing a creamy contrast.

Creamy Béchamel Sauce

½ medium onion, cut into chunks

1 cup water

¾ cup cooked or canned white beans, rinsed and drained

6 ounces reduced-fat firm silken tofu

1 tablespoon nutritional yeast flakes

1 teaspoon salt

¼ teaspoon dried garlic granules

Eggplant

3 pounds eggplant, cut into ¼"-thick slices

¾ cup fine dry bread crumbs

3 cups fat-free tomato-based pasta sauce

2 cups Creamy Béchamel Sauce

½ cup vegan Parmesan

For the sauce: Simmer the onion with 1 cup water in a medium saucepan, covered, for about 10 minutes. Place in a blender or food processor with the remaining ingredients and blend until very smooth. The sauce can be refrigerated in a covered container for up to 1 week.

For the eggplant: Arrange the eggplant slices in a single layer on a nonstick baking sheet. Broil 3" to 4" from the heat on both sides until lightly browned and soft inside (or grill on a nonstick indoor grill).

Preheat the oven to 325°F. Lay half of the eggplant in the bottom of a 10" round nonstick baking pan (or a baking pan lined with parchment) and top with half of the bread crumbs. Spread with half of the pasta sauce, béchamel sauce, and vegan Parmesan. Repeat with the remaining ingredients. Bake for 20 minutes, or until bubbly and browned on top.

MAKES 6 SERVINGS

Per serving: 262 calories, 11 g protein, 34 g carbohydrates, 7 g sugar, 1 g total fat, 6% calories from fat, 0 mg cholesterol, 10 g fiber, 697 mg sodium

Easy Veggie Fajitas

This restaurant favorite is easy to make at home.

     1 medium onion, cut into strips
    ¼ cup low-sodium vegetarian broth or water
     1 teaspoon ground cumin
     3 red, yellow, green, or mixed bell peppers, cored, seeded, and
       cut into strips
     2 cans (15 ounces each) black beans, drained and rinsed
     6 whole wheat tortillas (8" to 10")
     1 cup no-sugar-added tomato salsa

Steam-fry the onion in a large, heavy nonstick skillet until soft, adding very small amounts of broth or water as needed to prevent sticking and burning. Add the cumin and bell peppers and cook over medium heat until the peppers are tender. Heat the beans on high in the microwave for 1 minute.

Place a tortilla in a large, heavy skillet over medium-low heat. Add ½ cup of the beans and ½ cup of the onion mixture. Fold the tortilla in half over the filling and cook for 3 minutes. Repeat with the remaining tortillas and filling. Top with salsa and serve.

MAKES 6 SERVINGS

Per serving: 257 calories, 13 g protein, 50 g carbohydrates, 8 g sugar, 2 g total fat, 7% calories from fat, 0 mg cholesterol, 11 g fiber, 408 mg sodium

Recipe by Jennifer Reilly, RD

Sides

Orange Couscous Pilaf

Couscous looks like a grain but is actually a type of semolina pasta that cooks quickly and makes a delicious side dish.

    2   cups low-sodium vegetarian broth
    1   cup couscous
    1   cup grated carrots
    2   large oranges, peeled and cut into small chunks
    4   teaspoons grated orange peel
    2   tablespoons raisins
    ¼   teaspoon salt
    ¼   teaspoon ground cinnamon

Bring the broth and couscous to a boil in a large saucepan over high heat. Add the carrots, oranges, orange peel, raisins, salt, and cinnamon. Return to a boil, then turn off the heat, cover, and let stand for 10 minutes or until all liquid is absorbed. Fluff with a fork.

MAKES 4 SERVINGS

Per serving: 238 calories, 7 g protein, 52 g carbohydrates, 4 g sugar, 1 g total fat, 2% calories from fat, 0 mg cholesterol, 7 g fiber, 143 mg sodium

Brussels Sprouts with Lemon and Vegetarian Bacon

This is a delicious and quick brussels sprout dish. You can partially cook the sprouts ahead of time, stop the cooking with ice water, and then assemble and stir-fry the dish in minutes just before serving.

3 pounds brussels sprouts, trimmed and halved vertically
1 cup chopped vegetarian bacon (about 8 slices), such as Yves
   Veggie Canadian Bacon or Lightlife Fakin' Bacon
4 scallions, chopped
¼ cup low-sodium vegetarian broth
   Salt to taste
   Freshly ground black pepper to taste
2 tablespoons lemon juice

Add the brussels sprouts to a saucepan of boiling water and cook for 3 minutes. Drain immediately and plunge into ice-cold water to stop the cooking process. When they are cold, drain well.

Heat a large nonstick skillet, wok, or stir-fry pan over high heat. Add the bacon and scallions and steam-fry until the scallions are soft, adding very small amounts of water as needed to prevent sticking and burning. Add the sprouts and broth and stir-fry for about 3 minutes. Season with the salt and pepper and drizzle with the lemon juice. Toss and serve immediately.

MAKES 8 SERVINGS

Per serving: 71 calories, 12 g protein, 5 g carbohydrates, 1 g sugar, 0.5 g total fat, 6% calories from fat, 0 mg cholesterol, 2 g fiber, 331 mg sodium

Bulgur Wheat and Quinoa Pilaf

This is a tasty side dish for any meal.

- 1   cup bulgur wheat
- 1   cup quinoa
- 1   large onion, chopped
- 1   cup chopped celery
- 4   cups low-sodium vegetarian broth
- ¼   cup minced fresh parsley
- 1   teaspoon crushed dried rosemary or dried thyme or oregano
  Salt to taste

Place the bulgur and quinoa in a dry heavy skillet (such as cast-iron), stir-fry pan, or wok over high heat and cook, stirring constantly, until the grain smells toasty. Remove from the heat immediately and set aside.

Steam-fry the onion and celery in a large nonstick saucepan with a tight lid until the onion begins to soften. Add the broth, bulgur, quinoa, parsley, and rosemary, thyme, or oregano. Bring to a boil over high heat, then reduce the heat to low and cook, covered, for 20 minutes. Let stand for 5 minutes. Fluff with a fork and season with the salt.

MAKES 8 SERVINGS

Per serving: 174 calories, 6 g protein, 36 g carbohydrates, 1 g sugar, 2 g total fat, 7% calories from fat, 0 mg cholesterol, 6 g fiber, 46 mg sodium

Broccoli Stir-Fry in Black Bean Sauce

This is a colorful, quick, and fiber-rich accompaniment to any Asian-style meal.

  1   teaspoon minced or grated fresh ginger
  2   teaspoons crushed garlic
  2   tablespoons Chinese black bean sauce
  1   bunch broccoli
  1   large onion, cut into 6 wedges and layers separated
  2   tablespoons water
  3   tablespoons dry sherry or nonalcoholic sweet wine, such as
        Riesling
 1½ teaspoons cornstarch dissolved in ½ cup cold water

Mash the ginger and garlic together in a small bowl. Add the black bean sauce and mix well.

Divide the broccoli florets into bite-size pieces. Peel and chop the stems into ½" pieces and stir-fry with the florets and onion in a medium skillet over high heat. Add 2 tablespoons water, cover, and cook for 4 to 5 minutes or just until the broccoli is crisp-tender (add a little more water if necessary).

Add the ginger mixture, sherry or wine, and cornstarch mixture and stir until the sauce is thickened. Serve immediately.

MAKES 4 SERVINGS

Per serving: 85 calories, 6 g protein, 15 g carbohydrates, 1 g sugar, 1 g total fat, 4% calories from fat, 0 mg cholesterol, 0.5 g fiber, 416 mg sodium

Roasted Sweet Potatoes with Moroccan Spices

These sweet potatoes are easy to prepare, but your guests don't have to know that. The seeds add crunch as well as spice.

1½ pounds orange-fleshed sweet potatoes, peeled, halved
        lengthwise, and cut crosswise into ½" slices
¼ cup fat-free Italian dressing
1 tablespoon maple syrup
1½ teaspoons grated lemon peel
1½ teaspoons coriander seeds
1½ teaspoons cumin seeds
1½ teaspoons mustard seeds
    Salt to taste
    Freshly ground black pepper to taste

Position a rack in the bottom third of the oven and preheat the oven to 375°F.

Toss the sweet potatoes, dressing, maple syrup, lemon peel, and coriander, cumin, and mustard seeds together in a heavy nonstick rimmed baking sheet or shallow baking pan, then spread evenly in a shallow layer. Sprinkle with salt and pepper. Roast until tender and golden brown, stirring occasionally, for 30 to 45 minutes. Serve hot.

MAKES 5 SERVINGS

Per serving: 145 calories, 3 g protein, 33 g carbohydrates, 9 g sugar, 1 g total fat, 3% calories from fat, 0 mg cholesterol, 5 g fiber, 233 mg sodium

Roasted Green Beans, Fennel, Red Pepper, and Cauliflower with Dill

This is a delicious, easy, and colorful vegetable presentation.

2   medium fennel bulbs, tops cut off, halved, trimmed, and sliced
1   medium cauliflower, trimmed, broken into florets, and sliced
2   large red bell peppers, cored, seeded, and thickly sliced
6   cups fresh green beans, trimmed, or frozen whole young
       green beans
½   cup fat-free Italian dressing
2   tablespoons lemon juice
2   teaspoons dried dill weed or 2 tablespoons chopped fresh dill
1   teaspoon dried garlic granules
¼   cup chopped fennel leaves
     Salt to taste
     Freshly ground black pepper to taste

Preheat the oven to 350°F. Combine the fennel bulbs, cauliflower, bell peppers, beans, dressing, lemon juice, dill, garlic granules, fennel leaves, salt, and black pepper in a single layer in a large, shallow nonstick baking pan (use two pans if necessary to keep the vegetables in 1 shallow layer).

Place the pan or pans on the bottom oven rack. Bake for about 40 minutes, stirring occasionally with a spatula, until the vegetables are tender and beginning to brown slightly. Serve hot.

MAKES 8 SERVINGS

Per serving: 85 calories, 4 g protein, 19 g carbohydrates, 6 g sugar, 0.5 g total fat, 3% calories from fat, 0 mg cholesterol, 7 g fiber, 254 mg sodium

Desserts

Chocolate-Dipped Strawberries

This treat gives you the taste of rich chocolate with the healthful goodness of fresh fruit. Wax Orchards fat-free, fruit-sweetened organic fudge toppings are available in most health food stores. They come in six varieties.

¼ cup Wax Orchards fudge topping
12 large fresh whole strawberries, cleaned, with stems

Heat the topping in a small saucepan just until softened. Divide equally into 2 small bowls. Hold the strawberries by the stem ends, dip in the topping, and enjoy!

MAKES 2 SERVINGS

Per serving: 125 calories, 1 g protein, 29 g carbohydrates, 23 g sugar, 1 g total fat, 5% calories from fat, 0 mg cholesterol, 4 g fiber, 41 mg sodium

Cranberry–Orange–Pear Granola Crisp

Cranberries, oranges, and pears are made for each other. Serve this crisp with Lemon Crème (page 239).

4 large firm ripe pears, peeled, cored, and thinly sliced
2½ cups cranberries, thawed if frozen
Juice and finely grated peel of 1 medium orange
¼ teaspoon salt
¼ teaspoon freshly grated nutmeg
¼ teaspoon ground ginger
¾ cup (6 ounces) thawed frozen pear or apple juice concentrate
   or mixed pear, apple, and peach juice concentrate
2 tablespoons cornstarch
2 cups reduced-fat granola (no more than 4 percent calories
   from fat), such as Health Valley)

Preheat the oven to 400°F. Combine the pears, cranberries, orange juice, orange peel, salt, nutmeg, and ginger in a large bowl. Stir the juice concentrate and cornstarch together in a small bowl. Immediately pour into the fruit mixture and blend well. Pour into a 2-quart nonstick baking dish (or a baking dish lined with parchment). Bake for 20 minutes. Remove from the oven and reduce the heat to 350°F. Stir the fruit mixture thoroughly and sprinkle the granola evenly on top. Bake for 20 to 30 minutes or until the fruit is soft. Serve warm.

MAKES 8 SERVINGS

Per serving: 201 calories, 3 g protein, 51 g carbohydrates, 27 g sugar, 1 g total fat, 2% calories from fat, 0 mg cholesterol, 7 g fiber, 101 mg sodium

Lemon Crème

This simply delicious crème can be used as a pudding or a topping for fruit or cake. All you need are three ingredients (you use the lemon peel and the juice) and your blender.

- 1 package (12.3 ounces) reduced-fat extra-firm silken tofu, crumbled
- ⅓ cup Grade A (light) maple syrup or agave nectar
- 3 tablespoons fresh lemon juice
- 1 tablespoon grated lemon peel

Blend the tofu, maple syrup or agave nectar, lemon juice, and lemon peel until very smooth in a blender or food processor (or place in a bowl and use a hand-held blender). Refrigerate in a covered container until chilled.

MAKES 1¾ CUPS (4 SERVINGS)

Per serving: 106 calories, 6 g protein, 20 g carbohydrates, 17 g sugar, 1 g total fat, 5% calories from fat, 0 mg cholesterol, 0.5 g fiber, 88 mg sodium

Variation

Lemon-Ginger Crème: Fold in ¼ cup finely minced crystallized ginger.

Pineapple Sherbet Pops

You can make this variation on a favorite summer treat with a blender and just six ingredients.

1 package (12.3 ounces) reduced-fat firm or extra-firm silken tofu
3 tablespoons agave nectar or ⅓ cup sugar
4 teaspoons lemon juice
¾ teaspoon vanilla extract
1 can (19 ounces) juice-packed unsweetened crushed pineapple
¼ teaspoon coconut extract

Place the tofu, agave nectar or sugar, lemon juice, vanilla, pineapple (with juice), and coconut extract in a blender and process until smooth. Pour into 18 small ice pop molds, insert sticks, and freeze until solid. To serve, dip the bottoms of the molds in hot water for a few seconds so the pops slide out easily.

MAKES 18 SERVINGS

Per popsicle: 30 calories, 2 g protein, 6 g carbohydrates, 6 g sugar, 0.5 g total fat, 4% calories from fat, 0 mg cholesterol, 0.5 g fiber, 19 mg sodium

Berry Mousse

This is so easy that it's hardly a recipe! Your blender does most of the work. This can be eaten as a pudding or used as a topping for fruit.

    1 package (12.3 ounces) reduced-fat extra-firm silken tofu, crumbled
 2¾ cups thawed frozen unsweetened berries of choice
    3 tablespoons sugar or 2 tablespoons agave nectar
    1 tablespoon berry liqueur (optional)

Blend the tofu, berries, sugar or agave nectar, and liqueur, if desired, in a blender or food processor until smooth. Spoon into 4 pudding dishes and refrigerate until chilled.

MAKES 4 SERVINGS

Per serving: 123 calories, 7 g protein, 24 g carbohydrates, 17 g sugar, 1 g total fat, 5% calories from fat, 0 mg cholesterol, 3 g fiber, 89 mg sodium

Orange-Applesauce Date Cake

This easy lunchbox cake is moist and delicious—and even better the next day. The applesauce replaces both eggs and fat.

> 1 cup unsweetened smooth applesauce
> 1 tablespoon lemon juice
> 2 tablespoons water
> 1 tablespoon grated orange peel
> 1 cup whole wheat pastry flour (not regular whole wheat flour)
> ½ cup brown sugar
> ¼ cup oat flour (oatmeal ground in a dry blender or electric coffee mill) or barley flour
> ½ teaspoon ground cinnamon
> ¼ teaspoon salt
> ⅛ teaspoon ground nutmeg
> ⅛ teaspoon ground allspice
> 1 teaspoon baking soda
> 1 cup chopped pitted dates

Preheat the oven to 350°F. Place the applesauce, lemon juice, and 2 tablespoons water in a small saucepan over medium heat and warm slowly. Add the orange peel.

Mix the pastry flour, brown sugar, oat or barley flour, cinnamon, salt, nutmeg, and allspice in a medium bowl.

Stir the baking soda into the applesauce mixture (it will foam up). Pour immediately into the flour mixture and stir briefly but thoroughly.

Add the dates and mix briefly. Scoop the batter into a nonstick 9" × 9" cake pan, smooth the top, and bake for 10 minutes. Reduce the heat to 325°F and bake for 25 to 30 minutes or until it tests done with a cake tester. Transfer to a rack and cool completely. Make 2 evenly spaced cuts through the cake vertically, then horizontally, to make 9 squares.

MAKES 9 SERVINGS

Per serving: 169 calories, 3 g protein, 41 g carbohydrates, 24 g sugar, 0.5 g total fat, 2% calories from fat, 0 mg cholesterol, 4 g fiber, 199 mg sodium

NOTES

INTRODUCTION

[1] A. S. Nicholson et al., "Toward Improved Management of NIDDM: A Randomized, Controlled, Pilot Intervention Using a Low-Fat, Vegetarian Diet," *Preventive Medicine* 29 (1999): 87–91.

[2] N. D. Barnard et al., "The Effects of a Low-Fat, Plant-Based Dietary Intervention on Body Weight, Metabolism, and Insulin Sensitivity," *American Journal of Medicine* 118 (2005): 991–97.

CHAPTER 1

[1] M. Knip et al., "Environmental Triggers and Determinants of Type 1 Diabetes," *Diabetes* 54, suppl 2 (December 2005): S125–36.

CHAPTER 2

[1] T. Kuzuya, "Prevalence of Diabetes Mellitus in Japan Compiled from Literature," *Diabetes Research and Clinical Practice* 24, suppl (1994): S15–21.

[2] H. P. Himsworth, "The Dietetic Factor Determining the Glucose Tolerance and Sensitivity to Insulin of Healthy Men," *Clinical Science* 2 (1935): 67–94.

[3] D. B. Stone and W. E. Connor, "The Prolonged Effects of a Low-Cholesterol, High-Carbohydrate Diet upon the Serum Lipids in Diabetic Patients," *Diabetes* 12 (1963): 127–32.

[4] J. W. Anderson and K. Ward, "High-Carbohydrate, High-Fiber Diets for Insulin-Treated Men with Diabetes Mellitus," *American Journal of Clinical Nutrition* 32 (1979): 2312–21.

[5] R. J. Barnard, T. Jung, and S. B. Inkeles, "Diet and Exercise in the Treatment of NIDDM: The Need for Early Emphasis," *Diabetes Care* 17 (1994): 1469–72.

[6] A. S. Nicholson et al., "Toward Improved Management of NIDDM: A Randomized, Controlled, Pilot Intervention Using a Low-Fat, Vegetarian Diet," *Preventive Medicine* 29 (1999): 87–91.

[7] N. D. Barnard et al., "The Effects of a Low-Fat, Plant-Based Dietary Intervention on Body Weight, Metabolism, and Insulin Sensitivity," *American Journal of Medicine* 118 (2005): 991–97.

[8] A. E. Bunner, C. L. Wells, J. Gonzales, U. Agarwal, E. Bayat, N. D. Barnard. A dietary intervention for chronic diabetic neuropathy pain: a randomized controlled pilot study. *Nutrition & Diabetes* 2015 May 26;5:e158. doi: 10.1038/nutd.2015.8.

[9] N. D. Barnard et al., "The Effects of a Low-Fat, Plant-Based Dietary Intervention on Body Weight, Metabolism, and Insulin Sensitivity," *American Journal of Medicine* 118 (2005): 991–97.

[10] I. M. Stratton, A. L. Adler, and H. A. Neil, "Association of Glycaemia with Macrovascular and Microvascular Complications of Type 2 Diabetes (UKPDS 35): Prospective Observational Study," *British Medical Journal* 321 (2000): 405–12.

[11] UK Prospective Diabetes Study (UKPDS) Group, "Effect of Intensive Blood-Glucose Control with Metformin on Complications in Overweight Patients with Type 2 Diabetes (UKPDS 34)," *Lancet* 352 (1998): 854–65.

[12] D. Ornish et al., "Can Lifestyle Changes Reverse Coronary Heart Disease?" *Lancet* 336 (1990): 129–33.

[13] ———, "Intensive Lifestyle Changes for Reversal of Coronary Heart Disease," *Journal of the American Medical Association* 280 (1998): 2001–7.

[14] Y. Yokoyama, K. Nishimura, N. D. Barnard, et al. Vegetarian diets and blood pressure: a meta-analysis. *JAMA International Medicine* 2014;174(4):577–87.

[15] K. F. Petersen et al., "Impaired Mitochondrial Activity in the Insulin-Resistant Offspring of Patients with Type 2 Diabetes," *New England Journal of Medicine* 350 (2004): 664–71.

[16] Ibid.

[17] L. M. Sparks et al., "A High-Fat Diet Coordinately Downregulates Genes Required for Mitochondrial Oxidative Phosphorylation in Skeletal Muscle," *Diabetes* 54 (2005): 1926–33.

[18] A. V. Greco et al, "Insulin Resistance in Morbid Obesity: Reversal with Intramyocellular Fat Depletion," *Diabetes* 52 (2002): 144–51.

[19] L. M. Goff et al., "Veganism and Its Relationship with Insulin Resistance and Intramyocellular Lipid," *European Journal of Clinical Nutrition* 59 (2005): 291–8.

CHAPTER 3

[1] D. M. Nathan et al. and the Diabetes Control and Complications Trial/Epidemiology of Diabetes Interventions and Complications (DCCT/EDIC) Study Research Group, "Intensive Diabetes Treatment and Cardiovascular Disease in Patients with Type 1 Diabetes," *New England Journal of Medicine* 353 (2005): 2643–53.

[2] Diabetes Control and Complications Trial Research Group, "The Effect of Intensive Treatment of Diabetes on the Development and Progression of Long-Term Complications in Insulin-Dependent Diabetes Mellitus," *New England Journal of Medicine* 329 (1993): 977–86.

[3] E. L. Knight et al., "The Impact of Protein Intake on Renal Function Decline in Women with Normal Renal Function or Mild Renal Insufficiency," *Annals of Internal Medicine* 138 (2003): 460–7.

[4] J. Karjalainen et al., "A Bovine Albumin Peptide as a Possible Trigger of Insulin-Dependent Diabetes Mellitus," *New England Journal of Medicine* 327 (1992): 302–7.

[5] A. C. Alting, R. G. J. M. Meijer, and E. C. H. van Beresteijn, "Incomplete Elimination of the ABBOS Epitope of Bovine Serum Albumin under Simulated Gastrointestinal Conditions of Infants," *Diabetes Care* 20 (1997): 875–80.

[6] D. Hammond-McKibben and H. M. Dosch, "Cow's Milk, Bovine Serum Albumin, and IDDM: Can We Settle the Controversies?" *Diabetes Care* 20 (1997): 897–901.

[7] Ibid.

[8] American Academy of Pediatrics Work Group on Cow's Milk Protein and Diabetes Mellitus, "Infant Feeding Practices and Their Possible Relationship to the Etiology of Diabetes Mellitus," *Pediatrics* 94 (1994): 752–4.

[9] H. K. Akerblom et al., "Dietary Manipulation of Beta Cell Autoimmunity in Infants at Increased Risk of Type 1 Diabetes: A Pilot Study," *Diabetologia* 48 (2005): 829–37.

[10] P. S. Clyne and A. Kulczycki Jr. Human breast milk contains bovine IgG: relationship to infant colic?" *Pediatrics* 87 (1991): 439–44.

[11] K. Sadeharju et al., "Enterovirus Infections as a Risk Factor for Type 1 Diabetes: Virus Analyses in a Dietary Intervention Trial," *Clinical and Experimental Immunology* 132 (2003): 271–7.

CHAPTER 4

[1] L. M. Goff et al., "Veganism and Its Relationship with Insulin Resistance and Intramyocellular Lipid," *European Journal of Clinical Nutrition* 59 (2005): 291–8.

[2] E.C. Rizos, E.E. Ntzani, E. Bika, et al. Association between omega-3 fatty acid supplementation and risk of major cardiovascular disease events. *JAMA.* 2012;308:1024-33.

[3] S. M. Kwak, S. K. Myung, Y. J. Lee, H. G. Seo; Korean Meta-analysis Study Group... Efficacy of omega-3 fatty acid supplements (eicosapentaenoic acid and docosahexaenoic acid) in the secondary prevention of cardiovascular disease. *Archives of Internal Medicine* 2012; 172(9):686–94.

[4] S. Tonstad, T. Butler, R. Yan, G. E. Fraser. Type of vegetarian diet, body weight, and prevanence of type 2 diabetes. *Diabetes Care.* 2009;32:791–96.

[5] M. Kaushik, D. Mozaffarian, D. Spiegelman, et al. Long-chain omega-3 fatty acids, fish intake, and the risk of type 2 diabetes mellitus. *American Journal of Clinical Nutrition* 2009;90:613–20; N. D. Barnard, J. Cohen, D. J. Jenkins, et al. A low-fat, vegan diet improves glycemic control and cardiovascular risk factors in a randomized clinical trial in individuals with type 2 diabetes. *Diabetes Care* 2006;29:1777–83.

[6] N. D. Barnard, J. Cohen, D. J. Jenkins, G. Turner-McGrievy, L. Gloede, B. Jaster, K. Seidl, A. A. Green, S. Talpers. A low-fat, vegan diet improves glycemic control and cardiovascular risk factors in a randomized clinical trial in individuals with type 2 diabetes. *Diabetes Care* 2006;29:1777–83.

[7] Y. Papanikolaou et al., "Bean Consumption by Adults Is Associated with a More Nutrient Dense Diet and a Reduced Risk of Obesity," presented at the Experimental Biology Conference, April 1–5, 2006, San Francisco, CA.

[8] V. L. Fulgoni et al., "Bean Consumption by Children Is Associated with Better Nutrient Intake and Lower Body Weights and Waist Circumferences," presented at the Experimental Biology Conference, April 1–5, 2006, San Francisco, CA.

[9] S. J. Kim, R. J. de Souza, V. L. Choo, et al. Effect of dietary pulse consumption on body weight : a systematic review and meta-analysis of randomized controlled trials. Am J Clin Nutr;2016:103:1213-23.

[10] V. Ha, J. L. Sievenpiper, R. J. de Souza, et al. Effect of dietary pulse intake on established lipid targets for cardiovascular risk reduction: a systematic review and meta-analysis of randomized controlled trials. Canad Med Asso J. 2014;186:E252-62.

[11] D. G. Bailey, G. Dresser, M. O. Arnold. Grapefruit-medicaitonn interactions: forbidden fruit or avoidable consequences? CMAJ. 2013;185:309-16.

[12] E. L. Knight et al., "The Impact of Protein Intake on Renal Function Decline in Women with Normal Renal Function or Mild Renal Insufficiency," *Annals of Internal Medicine* 138 (2003): 460–7.

[13] E. Giovannucci et al., "Calcium and Fructose Intake in Relation to Risk of Prostate Cancer," *Cancer Research* 58 (1998): 442–7.

[14] J. M. Chan et al., "Dairy Products, Calcium, and Prostate Cancer Risk in the Physicians' Health Study," *American Journal of Clinical Nutrition* 74 (2001): 549–54.

[15] X. Gao, M. P. LaValley, K. L. Tucker. Prospective studies of dairy product and calcium intakes and prostate cancer risk: a meta-analysis. *Journal of the National Cancer Institute* 2005 Dec 7;97(23):1768–77.

[16] K. M. Wilson, E. L. Giovannucci, L. A. Mucci. Lifestyle and dietary factors in the prevention of lethal prostate cancer. *Asian Journal of Andrology.* 2012;14:265–74.

[17] H. L. Newmark, R. P. Heaney. Dairy products and prostate cancer risk. *Nutrition and Cancer* 2010;62(3):297–99.

[18] S. C. Larsson, N. Orsini, and A. Wolk, "Milk, Milk Products and Lactose Intake and Ovarian Cancer Risk: A Meta-Analysis of Epidemiological Studies," *International Journal of Cancer* 118 (2006): 431–41.

[19] J. M. Genkinger et al., "Dairy Products and Ovarian Cancer: A Pooled Analysis of 12 Cohort Studies," *Cancer Epidemiology Biomarkers & Prevention* 15 (2006): 364–72.

[20] B. Qin, P. G. Moorman, A. J. Alberg, et al. Dairy, calcium, vitamin D and ovarian cancer risk in African-American women. *British Journal of Cancer* 2016; 2016;115(9):1122–30.

[21] D. J. Jenkins et al., "Glycemic Index of Foods: A Physiological Basis for Carbohydrate Exchange," *American Journal of Clinical Nutrition* 34 (1981): 362–6.

[22] Ibid.

[23] J. Brand-Miller et al., "Low-Glycemic Index Diets in the Management of Diabetes," *Diabetes Care* 26 (2003): 2261–7.

[24] N. C. Howarth, E. Saltzman, and S. B. Roberts, "Dietary Fiber and Weight Regulation," *Nutrition Reviews* 59 (2001): 129–39.

25 N. D. Barnard et al., "The Effects of a Low-Fat, Plant-Based Dietary Intervention on Body Weight, Metabolism, and Insulin Sensitivity," *American Journal of Medicine* 118 (2005): 991–97.

26 M. G. Crane and C. Sample," "Regression of Diabetic Neuropathy with Total Vegetarian (Vegan) Diet," *Journal of Nutritional Medicine* 4 (1994): 431–9.

27 A. E. Bunner, C. L. Wells, J. Gonzales, U. Agarwal, E. Bayat, N. D. Barnard. A dietary intervention for chronic diabetic neuropathy pain: a randomized controlled pilot study. *Nutrition & Diabetes* 2015 May 26;5:e158. doi: 10.1038/nutd.2015.8.

28 G. M. Turner-McGrievy, et al. Effects of a low-fat, vegan diet and a step II diet on macro- and micronutrient intakes in overweight, postmenopausal women, *Nutrition* 20 (2004): 738–46.

29 E. L. Knight et al., "The Impact of Protein Intake on Renal Function Decline in Women with Normal Renal Function or Mild Renal Insufficiency," *Annals of Internal Medicine* 138 (2003): 460–7.

30 V. Melina, W. Craig, S. Levin. Position of the Academy of Nutrition and Dietetics: vegetarian diets. *Journal of the Academy of Nutrition and Dietetics* 2016;116:1970–80.

31 E. C. Westman et al. Effect of a 6-month adherence to a very low carbohydrate diet program. *American Journal of Medicine* 113 (2002): 30–36.

CHAPTER 6

1 N. D. Barnard et al., "The Effects of a Low-Fat, Plant-Based Dietary Intervention on Body Weight, Metabolism, and Insulin Sensitivity," *American Journal of Medicine* 118 (2005): 991–97.

2 N. C. Howarth, E. Saltzman, and S. B. Roberts, "Dietary Fiber and Weight Regulation," *Nutrition Reviews* 59 (2001): 129–39.

3 Barnard et al., "The Effects of a Low-Fat, Plant-Based Dietary Intervention."

4 J. A. Vernarelli, D. C. Mitchell, B. J. Rolls, T. J. Hartman. Dietary energy density is associated with obesity and other biomarkers of chronic disease in US adults. *European Journal Nutrition* 2015;54:59–65.

5 A. M. Dattilo and P. M. Kris-Etherton, "Effects of Weight Reduction on Blood Lipids and Lipoproteins: A Meta-Analysis," *American Journal of Clinical Nutrition* 56 (1992): 320–8.

6 E. C. Westman et al., "Effect of a 6-Month Adherence to a Very Low Carbohydrate Diet Program," *American Journal of Medicine* 113 (2002): 30–6.

7 W. S. Yancy et al., "A Low-Carbohydrate, Ketogenic Diet versus a Low-Fat Diet to Treat Obesity and Hyperlipidemia," *Annals of Internal Medicine* 130 (2004): 769–77.

8 E. L. Knight et al., "The Impact of Protein Intake on Renal Function Decline in Women with Normal Renal Function or Mild Renal Insufficiency," *American Journal of Medicine* 118 (2005): 460–7.

9 J. Coresh et al., "Prevalence of Chronic Kidney Disease and Decreased Kidney Function in the Adult US Population: Third National Health and Nutrition Examination Survey," *American Journal of Kidney Diseases* 41 (2003): 1–12.

10 K. D. Hall, T. Bemis, R. Brychta, et al. Calorie for calorie, dietary fat restriction results in more body fat loss than carbohydrate restriction in people with obesity. *Cell Metabolism.* 2015;22:427–36.

CHAPTER 7

1 G. B. Bolli and J. E. Gerich, "The 'Dawn Phenomenon'—A Common Occurrence in Both Non-Insulin-Dependent and Insulin-Dependent Diabetes Mellitus," *New England Journal of Medicine* 310 (1984): 746–50.

2 E. Selvin et al., "Meta-analysis: A1C and Cardiovascular Disease in Diabetes Mellitus," *Annals of Internal Medicine* 141 (2004): 421–31.

3 National Cholesterol Education Program, "Third Report of the National Cholesterol Education Program (NCEP) Expert Panel on Detection, Evaluation, and Treatment of High Blood Cholesterol in Adults (Adult Treatment Panel III) Final Report," *Circulation* 106 (2002): 3143–421.

[4] S. M. Grundy, et al. "Implications of Recent Clinical Trials for the National Cholesterol Education Program Adult Treatment Panel III Guidelines," *Circulation* 110 (2004): 227–39.

[5] American Diabetes Association, 2017

CHAPTER 9

[1] M. R. Yeomans et al., "Effects of Nalmefene on Feeding in Humans," *Psychopharmacology* 100 (1990): 426–32.

[2] D. J. Jenkins et al., "Low-Glycemic Index Diet in Hyperlipidemia: Use of Traditional Starchy Foods," *American Journal of Clinical Nutrition* 46 (1987): 66–71.

CHAPTER 10

[1] J. Hlebowicz, A. Hlebowicz, S. Lindstedt, et al. Effects of 1 and 3 g cinnamon on gastric emptying, satiety, and postprandial blood glucose, insulin, glucose-dependent insulinotropic polypeptide, glucagon-like peptide 1, and ghrelin concentrations in healthy subjects. *American Journal of Clinical Nutrition* 2009; 89:815–21.

[2] R. M. van Dam, F. B. Hu, L. Rosenberg, S. Krishnan, J. R. Palmer. Dietary calcium and magnesium, major food sources, and risk of type 2 diabetes in U.S. black women. *Diabetes Care* 2006 Oct;29(10):2238–43.

[3] W. Mertz, "Chromium Occurrence and Function in Biological Systems," *Physiological Reviews* 49 (1969): 163–239.

[4] K. N. Jeejeebhoy et al., "Chromium Deficiency, Glucose Intolerance, and Neuropathy Reversed by Chromium Supplementation in a Patient Receiving Long-Term Total Parenteral Nutrition," *American Journal of Clinical Nutrition* 30 (1977): 531–8.

[5] G. W. Landman, H. J. Bilo, S. T. Houweling, N. Kleefstra. Chromium does not belong in the diabetes treatment arsenal: current evidence and future perspectives. *World Journal of Diabetes* 2014;5:160–64.

[6] S. Jacob et al., "Oral Administration of RAC-Alpha-Lipoic Acid Modulates Insulin Sensitivity in Patients with Type-2 Diabetes Mellitus: A Placebo-Controlled Pilot Trial," *Free Radical Biology & Medicine* 27 (1999): 309–14.

[7] D. Ziegler, P. A. Low, W. J. Litchy, et al. Efficacy and safety of antioxidant treatment with α-lipoic acid over 4 years in diabetic polyneuropathy: the NATHAN 1 trial. *Diabetes Care* 2011;34(9):2054–60.

CHAPTER 11

[1] W. C. Knowler et al., "Reduction in the Incidence of Type 2 Diabetes with Lifestyle Intervention or Metformin," *New England Journal of Medicine* 346 (2002): 393–403.

[2] D. E. Thomas, E. J. Elliott, G. A. Naughton. Exercise for type 2 diabetes mellitus. *Cochrane Database System Review* 2006 Jul 19;(3):CD002968.

[3] N. G. Boulé et al., "Effects of Exercise on Glycemic Control and Body Mass in Type 2 Diabetes Mellitus: A Meta-Analysis of Controlled Clinical Trials," *Journal of the American Medical Association* 286 (2001): 1218–27.

[4] G. Hu et al., "Physical Activity, Cardiovascular Risk Factors, and Mortality among Finnish Adults with Diabetes," *Diabetes Care* 28 (2005): 799–805.

[5] ———, "Leisure Time, Occupational, and Commuting Physical Activity and the Risk of Stroke," *Stroke* 36 (2005): 1994–9.

[6] Diabetes Research in Children Network (DirecNet) Study Group. The effects of aerobic exercise on glucose and counterregulatory hormone concentrations in children with type 1 diabetes. *Diabetes Care* 29 (2006): 20–25.

CHAPTER 12

[1] N. D. Barnard, L. W. Scherwitz, and D. Ornish. "Adherence and Acceptability of a Low-Fat, Vegetarian Diet among Patients with Cardiac Disease," *Journal of Cardiopulmonary Rehabilitation* 12 (1992): 423–31.

[2] D. Ornish et al., "Can Lifestyle Changes Reverse Coronary Heart Disease?" *Lancet* 336 (1990): 129–33.

[3] ———, "Intensive Lifestyle Changes for Reversal of Coronary Heart Disease."

[4] N. D. Barnard, A. Akhtar, and A. Nicholson, "Factors That Facilitate Compliance to Lower Fat Intake," *Archives of Family Medicine* 4 (1995): 153–8.

[5] C. B. Esselstyn Jr., "Updating a 12-Year Experience with Arrest and Reversal Therapy for Coronary Heart Disease (an Overdue Requiem for Palliative Cardiology)," *American Journal of Cardiology* 84 (1999): 339–41.

[6] D. J. Jenkins, A. Mirrahimi, K. Srichaikul, et al. Soy protein reduces serum cholesterol by both intrinsic and food displacement mechanisms. *Journal of Nutrition* 2010;140(12):2302S–2311S.

[7] P. M. Kris-Etherton, F. B. Hu, E. Ros, J. Sabaté. The role of tree nuts and peanuts in the prevention of coronary heart disease: multiple potential mechanisms. *Journal of Nutrition* 2008 Sep;138(9):1746s–1751s.

[8] D. J. Jenkins et al., "Direct Comparison of a Dietary Portfolio of Cholesterol-Lowering Foods with a Statin in Hypercholesterolemic Participants," *American Journal of Clinical Nutrition* 81 (2005): 380–7.

[9] A. Poobalan, L. Aucott, W. C. Smith, A. Avenell, R. Jung, J. Broom, A. M. Grant. Effects of weight loss in overweight/obese individuals and long-term lipid outcomes—a systematic review. *Obesity Review* 2004;5(1):43–50.

[10] S. Berkow and N. D. Barnard, "Blood Pressure Regulation and Vegetarian Diets," *Nutrition Reviews* 63 (2005): 1–8.

CHAPTER 13

[1] M. G. Crane, "Sample C. Regression of Diabetic Neuropathy with Total Vegetarian (Vegan) Diet," *Journal of Nutritional Medicine* 4 (1994): 431–9.

[2] D. Ziegler. Efficacy and safety of antioxidant treatment.

[3] D. F. Horrobin, "Essential Fatty Acids in the Management of Impaired Nerve Function in Diabetes," *Diabetes* 46, suppl 2 (1997): S90–93.

[4] A. A. Sima. Acetyl-L-carnitine in diabetic polyneuropathy: experimental and clinical data. *CNS Drugs* 2007;21 Suppl 1:13–23; discussion 45–6.

[5] I. De Leeuw et al., "Long Term Magnesium Supplementation Influences Favourably the Natural Evolution of Neuropathy in Mg-Depleted Type 1 Diabetic Patients (T1dm)," *Magnesium Research* 17 (2004): 109–14.

[6] M. Lu et al., "Prospective Study of Dietary Fat and Risk of Cataract Extraction among US Women," *American Journal of Epidemiology* 161 (2005): 948–59.

[7] N. Karas-Kuzelicki, V. Pfeifer, J. Lukac-Bajalo. Synergistic effect of high lactase activity genotype and galactose-1-phosphate uridyl transferase (GALT) mutations on idiopathic presenile cataract formation. *Clinical Biochemistry* 2008 Jul;41(10-11):869–74.

[8] L. Ma, X. M. Lin. Effects of lutein and zeaxanthin on aspects of eye health. *Journal of the Science of Food and Agriculture* 2010 Jan 15;90(1):2–12. doi: 10.1002/jsfa.3785.

[9] R. G. Cumming, P. Mitchell, and W. Smith, "Diet and Cataract: The Blue Mountains Eye Study," *Ophthalmology* 107 (2000): 450–6.

[10] M. S. Morris et al., "Moderate Alcoholic Beverage Intake and Early Nuclear and Cortical Lens Opacities," *Ophthalmic Epidemiology* 11 (2004): 53–65.

[11] L. Azadbakht, S. Atabak, A. Esmaillzadeh. Soy protein intake, cardiorenal indices, and C-reactive protein in type 2 diabetes with nephropathy: a longitudinal randomized clinical trial. *Diabetes Care* 2008 Apr;31(4):648–54.

[12] Y. Yokoyama, K. Nishimura, N. D. Barnard, et al. Vegetarian diets and blood pressure: a meta-analysis. *JAMA International Medicine* 2014;174(4):577–87.

INDEX

Underscored page references indicate sidebars and tables. **Boldface** references indicate illustrations.

A

Addictive foods, 132–35
  substitutes for, 137–38
Aerobic exercise, 149, 154, 155
Albumin testing, 110, 183
Alcohol avoidance
  for cataract prevention, 181
  for triglycerides reduction, 142
  with warfarin, 143
Alpha-linolenic acid, 57, 58, 72
Alpha-lipoic acid, 147, 178
American cuisine, 118
Amino acids, 69, 70, 134
Anemia, 71, 111
Animal fat
  calories in, 91–92
  composition of, 162, 163
Animal products
  eliminating
    for cholesterol reduction, 58, 164–65, 170
    in diabetes reversal diet, 17, 18, 19, 20, 42–48
    for heart health, 22
    for weight control, 92, 92, 126
  fat and cholesterol in, 30–31, 42–43, 44, 58, 65
Animal protein
  in breakfast foods, 76
  calcium loss from, 70, 71
  kidney damage from, 31, 46, 53, 55, 69–70, 98, 182
A1C. *See* Hemoglobin A1C
Appetite control, 95–97
Apples
  Breakfast Barley with Fruit, 197
  Red Cabbage Slaw with Cranberries and Apples, 224
Applesauce
  Orange-Applesauce Date Cake, 248
Artery blockages
  diet reversing, 161–62, 163–64
  diet worsening, 165

Artichoke hearts
  Cherry Tomato and Brown Rice Salad with Artichoke Hearts, 222
  Lemon and Artichoke Tagine (Moroccan Stew), 230–31
  Mediterranean Veggie Panini, 219
Artificial sweeteners, 137
Asparagus
  Asparagus and Veggie Ham Panini, 217
Atkins Diet, 71
Autonomic neuropathy, 176–77

B

Bacon, veggie. *See* Vegetarian bacon
Bacon grease, 162–63
Bagels, 76
Barley
  Barley and Winter Squash Chowder, 212
  Breakfast Barley with Fruit, 197
  fiber in, 168
  uses for, 87
Barley flour
  Tender Barley Cornbread, 201
Beans
  for appetite control, 96
  Black Bean Soft Tacos, 216–17
  Broccoli Stir-Fry in Black Bean Sauce, 241
  canned, 86
  cholesterol reduction from, 49, 168, 170–71
  Easy Veggie Fajitas, 237
  energy density of, 97
  fiber in, 113
  gas from, 49, 140–41
  nutrients in, 70, 71, 86
  Vegetarian Mixed-Bean Chili Express, 232–33
  Vegetarian "Refried" Beans, 205
  for weight control, 49
  White Bean and Sweet Potato Stew, 228
Beef
  cholesterol in, 44, 76, 164, 165
  fat in, 44, 45, 57, 91, 162, 163

255

Fat buildup, in muscle cells, 23–26, **24**, 28, 41, 60, 128
Fat burning, disabled by fatty foods, 26, 27
Fat-Free Oil Substitute, 208
Fatigue, as diabetes symptom, 3, 4
Fatty foods
    disabling fat burning, 26, 27
    eliminating, 74
Fennel
    Roasted Green Beans, Fennel, Red Pepper, and Cauliflower with Dill, 243
Fiber
    checking intake of, 93, 99, 112–13, 127–28
    for constipation prevention, 140
    for hunger prevention, 131
    soluble, 75, 86, 168, 170
    sources of, 93, 168
    for triglycerides reduction, 142
    weight loss from, 65, 75, 92–93, <u>92</u>, 99
Fight-or-flight response, 130
Fish, <u>44</u>, 45, 164
Fish oils, 45, 58
Flexibility exercises, 149
Food addictions
    categories of, 132–35
    causes of, 135–36, 138–40
    managing, 137–38
Food shopping, 85–86
Foot examination, 115, 178
Foot injuries, 155, 178
Fractures, 70, 71
Frozen meals, 81
Fruits. *See also specific fruits*
    for appetite control, 96
    for cholesterol protection, 169
    fiber in, 113
    on Power Plate, 50–51
    for satisfying sugar cravings, 137
    as snacks, 84, 88

G

Gamma-linolenic acid, 178
Gas-causing foods, 49, 140–41
Gastric bypass surgery, 27–28
Genes
    cravings influenced by, 138–40
    for fat burning, 26
    role of, in diabetes, 9, 28, 32
Gestational diabetes, 8, 101
GI. *See* Glycemic index
Glaucoma, 179
Glomerular filtration rate, 110
Glucose, function of, 3–4
Glucose tablets, 103, 104
Glucose testing, 101–5
Glucose testing equipment, 11–12
Glycemic index (GI), 58–62, 74. *See also* High-glycemic-index foods; Low-glycemic-index foods

Grains. *See* Whole grains
Granola
    Cranberry-Orange-Pear Granola Crisp, 244–45
Grapefruit, interacting with drugs, <u>50</u>
Green beans
    Low-Fat Guacamole, 204–5
    Roasted Green Beans, Fennel, Red Pepper, and Cauliflower with Dill, 243
Greens
    Black-Eyed Peas with Sweet Potatoes and Greens, 233
    BLT Salad, 226–27
    Italian Stuffed Griddle Dumplings (Consum), 218
    Mediterranean Veggie Panini, 219
    nutrients in, 70, 71
    Sautéed Portobello Mushroom Salad, 225
Grogan, Bryanna Clark, 191
Guacamole
    Low-Fat Guacamole, 204–5

H

Happy Cow's Vegetarian Guide, 120
HDL cholesterol, 30, 109, 172–73
Health care providers, role of, 184–87
Heart attacks, cause of, 161
Heart disease
    exercising with, 153
    reversing, 22–23, 31, 65, 161–68
Heart health
    exercise for, 150
    fish oils and, 45
Heart problems
    A1C and, 108
    LDL level and, 109
    preventing, in type 1 diabetes, 29
    risk factors for, 159–60
Hemoglobin A1C
    dopamine influencing, 140
    guidelines for, 107–8, 128
    in prediabetes, 8
    reducing
        with exercise, 150
        for heart health, 173
        with low-glycemic-index foods, 61–62
        with vegan diet, 21, 63, 175–76
    testing, <u>5</u>, 8, 107–8
High blood pressure, 109–10, 179, 182
High blood pressure medications, 14
High-glycemic-index foods, 59–60, 111–12, 133, 173
High-protein breakfast foods, 77–78
High-protein diets, 71, 98, <u>98</u>
Honey, <u>88</u>
Hummus, 80, 84, 87
    Spinach Hummus, 206–7
Hunger, 130–31, 136